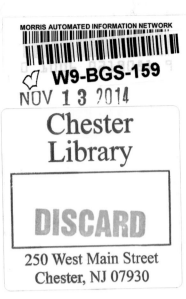
Your Cervix (Just) Has a Cold

Your Cervix
(Just) Has a Cold

The Truth About Abnormal Pap Smears & HPV

Dr. Brandie Gowey, NMD

NEW YORK

Your Cervix (Just) Has a Cold
The Truth About Abnormal Pap Smears & HPV

ISBN 978-1-61448-684-8 paperback
ISBN 978-1-61448-685-5 eBook
Library of Congress Control Number: 2013936638

Morgan James Publishing
The Entrepreneurial Publisher
5 Penn Plaza, 23rd Floor,
New York City, New York 10001
(212) 655-5470 office • (516) 908-4496 fax
www.MorganJamesPublishing.com

Cover Design by:
Rachel Lopez
www.r2cdesign.com

Interior Design by:
Bonnie Bushman
bonnie@caboodlegraphics.com

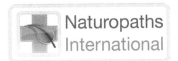

In an effort to support local communities, raise awareness and funds, Morgan James Publishing donates a percentage of all book sales for the life of each book to Habitat for Humanity Peninsula and Greater Williamsburg.

Get involved today, visit
www.MorganJamesBuilds.com.

Habitat
for Humanity®
Peninsula and
Greater Williamsburg
Building Partner

This book is dedicated to

My brother,
Jeremiah J. Gowey

August 20, 1982—June 28, 2010

I am always here for you Bro, your passing doesn't take that away.
I love you and miss you more than I can say.
I'd give anything to be able to go on just
one more motorcycle ride with you.

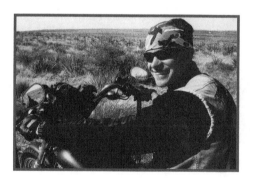

And to my patients,

who have always believed in me and in Naturopathic Medicine.
Thank you for trusting the process.

This book is for you and for your children.

United States of America

United States Patent and Trademark Office

GOWEY PROTOCOL

Reg. No. 4,174,827

Registered July 17, 2012

Int. Cl.: 1

TRADEMARK

PRINCIPAL REGISTER

DR. BRANDIE E. GOWEY, NMD (UNITED STATES INDIVIDUAL)
2532 N 4TH ST, #537
FLAGSTAFF, AZ 86004

FOR: PLANT EXTRACTS MADE FROM SARRACENIA PURPUREA AND OTHER CARNI-VOROUS PLANTS, USED IN THE MANUFACTURE OF TOPICAL GELS AND CREAMS FOR ANTI-MICROBIAL AND ANTI-VIRAL THERAPEUTIC USES, IN CLASS 1 (U.S. CLS. 1, 5, 6, 10, 26 AND 46).

FIRST USE 12-1-2009; IN COMMERCE 11-13-2011.

THE MARK CONSISTS OF STANDARD CHARACTERS WITHOUT CLAIM TO ANY PAR-TICULAR FONT, STYLE, SIZE, OR COLOR.

SER. NO. 85-471,325, FILED 11-13-2011.

JEFFREY LOOK, EXAMINING ATTORNEY

Director of the United States Patent and Trademark Office

Table of Contents

Acknowledgements

When I look back at the days and months leading up to the moment I took pen to paper, there are many who came across my path and helped me along the way in the process of writing this book. If I forget to mention anyone, it is not personal; please know you have my gratitude!

Thanks to...

Mom, for your never-ending support and belief that I can be successful. To my dad, for pushing me to be the best I could be when I was little. I will not forget those late night walks we did when I was young; I remember everything you said, Dad. I took notes!

The folks at Professional Compounding Centers of America (PCCA) of Houston, Texas. The staff at PCCA, especially Gus Bassani, was key for the development of the *Gowey Protocol®* *Gel*.

My Attorneys Quan Nguyen and Brian Harlow for helping me protect the *Gowey Protocol®*.

Dr. Bob Waters, PhD, who first asked me to "do something" with a plant extract: this extract I turned into the *Gowey Protocol®* and *Gowey Protocol®* *Gel*. I appreciate that you entrusted this particular plant to my care, and that you chose me because of my work with Naturopaths International (NI). The money from both the sale of this book and the *Gel* will go towards funding for NI (*naturopathsinternational. org*) as well as additional Naturopathic research.

Joel Osteen, for inspiring me every day. I love your sermons. Thank you!

Patients who participated in the clinical trials who tried the **Gel** for various applications, and who entrusted their health care to me.

Sherry Tackett, for sending me some of the first patients who worked through the **Gowey Protocol®**.

The pitcher plant for giving me this gift of healing to share, and to our Creator for planting the seed of desire in my heart to serve humanity.

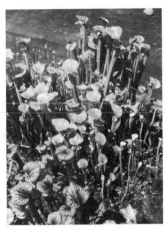

Sarracenia spp

Foreword

It has been decades since scientists discovered that the Human Papillomavirus (HPV) causes cervical cancer in women. When it was first identified, the treatments were harsh and quite invasive. The typical treatment usually consisted of either burning or freezing off the diseased tissue, which was quite painful and often did not work.

Naturopathic Physicians regarded this virus as an assault on the immune system. They were looking for ways to enhance the immune system rather than go to battle with it and cause more harm.

The author of this book, Dr. Brandie Gowey, has given us an opportunity to view the patient as a whole person when dealing with HPV or abnormal pap smears. Looking at the mind, body and spirit is the key to healing in all situations, especially with cervical diseases (or any disease). Her treatment for this elusive virus is multi-dimensional and, because of that, there is intense healing with the patient.

As a holistic nurse practitioner in women's health, I have learned a great deal from Dr. Gowey's teachings with her patients. Her research far exceeds any other work done on this topic. Dr. Gowey is not only compassionate about service to patients, she is also a dedicated Doctor of Naturopathy who will not stop her research until all women who have been affected by HPV can be offered the choice of sparing her cervix and healing within.

As a woman, I can relate to many of the stories shared in this book. I fell prey to the Human Papillomavirus (HPV) when I was in my twenties. I did not think I was susceptible to contracting a sexually transmitted disease because I am a lesbian; I did not realize that HPV could be transmitted from woman to woman contact. I was shocked when my female partner returned from her annual pap test and informed me that she had HPV. I found out later that she had "high-grade dysplasia" caused by HPV, and that it was pre-cancerous.

The physician recommended that I be tested right away. I was diagnosed with external condyloma, as well as mild dysplasia to my cervix. The physician recommended we both have a laser procedure done called LEEP. Even though it was many years ago, I still remember how devastated I was when told that I had a sexually transmitted disease that required an extensive laser procedure in an outpatient surgical facility. The experience was not pleasant.

They secured me down on a surgical table with my legs strapped to the stirrups. It was extremely uncomfortable as well as frightening. The surgical team walked in wearing protective eyewear. They looked like a group of aliens. They placed the eyewear on me as well, and then everything went blurry. I could hear them talking and the sound of the laser. When I woke up, I was very sore and could barely walk to the car. As the tissue starting sloughing off, I was in excruciating pain. I was given instructions to do sea salt soaks for the discomfort. Needless to say, I spent three days in the bathtub soaking away the pain, both physical and emotional. It has taken many years to heal psychologically from that experience. I experienced a lot of different emotions as a result of having HPV. I was sad about being betrayed by my partner. I was angry that I had not been aware of her sexual behaviors, and that I had not asked for this disease. I felt it important to share my experience with all who read this book in hopes that, whether you are straight, lesbian, gay, or bisexual, you will take precautions with any future sexual partners.

The information provided in this book will benefit all who read it, including patients, partners of patients, men, and physicians. It speaks for all of us who are dedicated in assisting others in their healing process. Enjoy it with great gratitude for the in-depth knowledge this author has on the subject. She has researched hard and long to develop this very special plant-based protocol now named the "*Gowey Protocol®*."

— *Sherry Tackett, WHNP*

Background

What is Naturopathic Medicine?

Most people I meet, when I mention I am a Naturopathic Physician, think I prescribe supplements and herbs instead of drugs. Not so.

A true Naturopathic Physician is a type of medical doctor who will do a full health history during your initial intake. Gathering this information usually takes at least an hour and, during that time, connections in your health that identify a root cause of symptoms will be identified. An individualized treatment plan is then designed to treat that root cause (or causes), which occasionally may involve the use of medications (for example, thyroid medication if your thyroid is low).

A good Naturopathic Physician will work with you on treatments and protocols that resonate with you, that get you better, and that help support you emotionally, mentally, physically and spiritually. If you find a great Naturopathic Physician to work with, I promise you will love the kind of medical care you receive.

All Naturopathic Physicians have what are called "modalities" that they offer. A list of example modalities include:

Acupuncture
Herbs
Homeopathy

Adjustments (Physical Manipulation)
Mind/Body Medicine
Vitamin I.V./I.V. Therapies
Injection Therapies (like Prolotherapy)
Supplement Counseling
Nutritional Counseling
Hydrotherapy
Genetic Testing

It is key for you to do some homework to find a physician you resonate with. If there is not a licensed Naturopath in your area, I'm sure you can find one (such as myself) to do phone consultations. Phone consultations can help guide you further in finding local help for your health concerns.

There are only a few medical schools offering Naturopathy as a specialty (and, yes, it is considered a medical specialty). A few of the top medical schools that offer this specialty are:

Bastyr University School of Naturopathic Medicine
(Seattle, WA)
Southwest College of Naturopathic Medicine
(Tempe, AZ)
National College of Naturopathic Medicine
(Portland, OR)
University of Bridgeport College of Naturopathic Medicine
(Bridgeport, CT)
Canadian College of Naturopathic Medicine
(Toronto, QB)

Naturopathic Physicians practice according to the following ideals and principles:

The Healing Power of Nature
Your body has the ability to heal itself, given the right nutrients and support.
First, Do No Harm
Find and utilize treatments that are safe, noninvasive, and have minimal risks.
Find the Cause

Identify and treat the causes of the disease or condition, do not treat the symptoms.

Treat the Whole Person

Everyone is unique and has different life experiences as well as biochemistry. Understanding this in each person allows the physician to develop individualized treatment plans.

Prevention as Cure

Preventing problems and disease before they start, understanding the patient well enough to help guide them in making choices and living wisely in a health-full way. True "wellness" medicine.

Introduction

I will **never forget** the very first patient I treated for an abnormal pap smear (pap). She was young, 21-years-old. She had waited for her first sexual experience to be with a man she thought loved her and was going to commit fully to her. She had waited, in part, because of her religious affiliations, but also because she wanted to be sure the man she would be with the first time cared and wanted what was best for her. However, after intercourse with him, she never heard from him again. She then started to worry about the possibility that she may have contracted a sexually transmitted disease, or that she was pregnant.

She was not pregnant, but her pap did come back as being pre-cancerous and she was positive for the Human Papillomavirus, a sexually transmitted virus known as HPV. It was very difficult for me to tell her she had contracted this virus, and that we now had to work together to prevent cancer.

Since that time, I have extended a Kleenex to dozens and dozens of women, all with similar stories about how they got HPV and their first abnormal pap smear. In medical school, I had learned that HPV was responsible for causing the pre-cancerous results. It was something to be greatly feared. There is such shame women feel in discovering their results are abnormal. Was it OK to continue to have sex with other partners? What if they pass the virus on to someone else? All were questions that needed to be answered and evaluated with honesty, care and compassion.

In working with my patients who had abnormal pap smears—and ultimately with the virus—I began to discover that the virus might be more of an opportunist rather than the cause of the problems. In my heart and mind, I began to open to the possibility that the virus takes advantage of a lack of wellness. And that lack of wellness leaves the cervix more vulnerable to HPV-related disease.

In this book, I share what I have learned from the work done with my patients and HPV. It is important for me to note that I am not claiming a cure. What I am doing is providing guidance and insight into the possibility that you may heal your body, even from something as scary as an abnormal pap result. It can happen all by the power of your will, determination, faith, and trust that your body knows how to heal if given the right nutrients and support.

It is estimated that over 50% of the world's female population has HPV: the statistic is higher in lower socioeconomic areas. If you are a woman living with HPV, I am here to tell you that you can be healthy! Your cervix literally has a cold, and you have nothing to be ashamed of. I developed what has become known as the "**Gowey Protocol®**" (named as such by Dr. Bob Waters, PhD, of Southwest College of Naturopathic Medicine, who was my professor of genetics and biochemistry), by working with patients who wanted treatments other than what is conventionally offered.

If you are a patient who has developed cancer from the effects of HPV on your cervix, I am not making light of your situation. I am offering education, options and preventative medicine for those with current pre-cancerous lesions.

For me, the **Gowey Protocol®** developed out of an amazing journey. With each patient whose health improved, I learned more. I developed a deep respect for the Human Papillomavirus and saw increasingly how everything in life is in such a delicate balance. Once you learn where your weakness is in terms of your health, you can change things for the better. It's very empowering!

With all the abnormal pap patients I cared for, I used a plant-based gel *(Gowey Protocol® Gel)* that's applied vaginally, via an applicator several nights a week by the patient and manually by the physician (at each monthly follow-up).

The **Gowey Protocol® Gel** is a proprietary blend of extracts of carnivorous plants (Sarracenia purpurea and flava) and antioxidants in an aloe vera base. One of these plants was historically used as an anti-viral against smallpox (Lancet 1862) and works well when combined with all the healthy choices and changes I explain in this book.

I want to mention that I do not feel you should do any of the treatments I suggest absent of working with a Naturopathic Physician trained in proper application of the **Gowey Protocol®**. Cervical dysplasia, while reversible, is still a pre-cancerous lesion and should be monitored. And, while I use the plant-based **Gel** on the cervix to aid in healing, you may have a practitioner who uses other applications such as suppositories. Through the years, I have gotten my work with women down to an art: I know quickly what their obstacle to cure is and what we need to do to make changes possible. I can train your physician in the full *Protocol*, but the responsibility for healing lies with you.

I also want to emphasize that the **Gowey Protocol**® treatment is not meant for everyone. If you are not ready in your heart to completely commit to your health, the full **Gowey Protocol**® treatment is not for you, and there is nothing wrong with that. I am confident there are things in this book that you can still take with you and implement into your life. In my experience, patients who have a strong body/mind connection, or who are working towards that, have the best outcomes.

Chapter One

What is an Abnormal Pap?

Your cervix—the lower part of your uterus that dilates during labor, thereby allowing birth—has a thin layer of cells on its surface. This layer has two kinds of cells: one called columnar, in the shape of a column; and the other called squamous, meaning flat. Where these two cells meet is where abnormal cell changes occur, and it is where a physician takes a sample of cells during your annual pap exam.

This junction of cells is where a virus, the Human Papillomavirus (HPV), can be active. This virus is sexually transmitted, and has been established in all the medical standards of care and literature as "the cause" (*mdconsult.com/cervicaldysplasia*) of pre-cancerous changes in the cervix. These changes in cells become termed "dysplastic", or pre-cancerous, if an abnormal result shows in your pap. There are various levels of this dysplasia that, if left untreated, can lead to cervical cancer (*nlm.nih.gov*). In 2001, there were 4,400 deaths due to cervical cancer in the U.S., with 12,000 newly diagnosed cases. Worldwide, there are 530,000 new cases of cervical cancer annually (Fonseca-Moutinho 2011). Incidences tend to be higher in Hispanic populations (*mdconsult.com/cervicaldysplasia*).

Dysplasia (pre-cancer) is graded in several steps before it is considered cancer:

1. *Atypical Cells of Undetermined Significance (ASGUS)*: This basically means there is a problem but many practitioners choose to watch and wait to

1

see what happens (generally re-paping within six months). For some women, ASGUS may resolve back to normal tissues. The conventional medical community calls this "spontaneous resolution", having no explanation as to why or how this happens (*mdconsult.com/cervicaldysplasia*).

2. *Low-Grade Intraepithelial Lesion (LSIL)*: This means you are three steps (mild dysplasia) away from cancer. Cells are becoming increasingly abnormal. Cells are often graded as CIN I (cervical intraepithelial neoplasia, grade one).

3. *High-Grade Intraepithelial Lesion (HSIL)*: This means you are one to two steps away from cancer (CIN II or III, cervical intraepithelial neoplasia, grade two and three).

The course of treatment varies with the opinion and experience of your gynecologist (GYN). Most physicians will conduct another pap in six months if you are ASGUS and hysterectomy or LEEP/cryotherapy if you have more advanced stages (LSIL or HSIL) after a biopsy (colposcopy) is performed. LEEP (loop electrosurgical excision procedure) is the most common procedure; it involves the use of heat to sear the cells that are abnormal on the cervix. Cryotherapy involves the use of cold to sear the cells, and hysterectomy is surgical removal of your uterus and cervix.

The problem with some of these procedures is the risk factor(s). With LEEP alone, there is an increased risk of pre-term delivery, premature rupture of membranes prior to delivery, and low birth weight infants (Sanson et al. 2005). I usually see scar tissue develop on or over the cervix after a LEEP.

The exact percentages of women with HPV are unknown, with estimates at 50% or greater (*emedicinehealth.com*) of the global population. While men are generally thought to be carriers, they do not usually have symptoms other than genital warts, although they can also develop cancer from HPV.

While experts and the physician standard of care agree, and while, as doctors, we are taught that HPV is the cause of abnormal paps, it has been widely published in studies and hypothesized (by myself included) that there are risk factors contributing to the cervical lesions because, in some cases, regression of viral activity has been documented (Trimble et al. 2005).

In my work treating patients with histories of abnormal pap smears, I do not feel the virus is the cause. I feel the virus is the opportunist of deeper problems and pathologies. Some are treatable (i.e., dietary changes), and some are difficult or not treatable with our current technologies (i.e., genetics). Fenseca et al. (2011) agrees with me:

HPV has been the strongest epidemiologic factor associated with intraepithelial neoplasia and cancer of the cervix, and is considered a necessary cause but is not sufficient as cause of cervical dysplasia.

The virus is opportunistic. It takes advantage of a susceptible cervical cell lining. However, after going through my treatment protocol, most of my patients have not had repeat abnormal paps, even though they still have the virus. And, if they do get a recurrence of the abnormality, it's because they slid back into old patterns, had large amounts of external stressors that made them more susceptible, or they got a new strain of HPV. There are over 80 strains of HPV, 20 of which have been identified as "cancer-causing".

I worked closely with hundreds of patients from 2009 to 2012, all with varying degrees of abnormal pap smears; some with newly diagnosed paps and others with repeat dysplasia. I started to keep records of the causes I was seeing and then did an extensive literature review. I found confirmation for all of my findings already known and studied within the research. The risk factors of cervical dysplasia and cancer are:

1. *Stress:* Studies have shown that women who perceive stress higher than other women have a "non-response" to HPV-16 (the most cancer-causing form of the virus). This means T cells (the type of immune cell that responds to viruses) do not respond to the presence of the virus (Fang 2008). Dr. Walter Crinnion, NMD, would say the inactivity of T cells is in part due to environmental toxicities or abnormal mitochondrial function (Crinnion 2012).

2. *Birth Control Pills (OCP):* Study after study demonstrates a positive correlation between OCP use and cervical dysplasia (McFarlande-Anderdone et al. 2008).

3. *Co-Infection with Other Viruses, such as HIV/AIDS:* HIV is associated with a significantly high risk of cervical dysplasia (Firnhaber 2009).

4. *Cigarette Smoking:* Direct link to toxins in cigarette smoke adhering to cervical cells (Fenseca et al. 2011).

5. *Suppression of Immune System:* Lower T cell response equals higher risk (Bipin et al. 2010).

6. *Genetics (genetic marker CCR2):* Women with this marker may develop cervical dysplasia independent of HPV (Chatterjec et al. 2010).

7. *Gene Deletions in Detoxification Pathways*: Changes in groupings of enzymes that normally help us detoxify toxins has been linked to cervical dysplasia/cancer, specifically in pathways named CYP1A1, GSTM1, GSTT (Goodman et al. 2001).

8. *Nutritional Status*: Low folate, vitamin A, vitamin C and antioxidant levels are linked to dysplasia (Marshall 2003).

9. *Medication Use*: Especially from drugs that affect hormones (Marshall 2003).

10. *Lack of Vaccinations*: The current vaccine targets only two subtypes of HPV (16 and 18; Lehtinen et al. 2012), ignoring the other 18 that are "cancer-producing".

11. *Excessive Acidity*: Acidity of body tissues robs you of nutrients to fight cancerous lesions (Aihara 1986).

12. *Sugar in Diet*: One teaspoon of sugar suppresses your immune system for four to six hours, leading to inflammation (which I learned in medical school) and have seen this clinically.

13. *Emotional Health*: What you say actually happens (Osteen 2011), so be careful about the words you send out. If you believe the virus will cause cancer, it will.

14. *Alcohol/Drug Abuse*: Drugs rob your body of nutrients, because of the nutrients required to break them down once ingested (Fenseca et al. 2011).

15. *Food Sensitivities*: These cause chronic inflammation that starts at your gut and can spread to other tissues/organs (clinical observation).

16. *Environmental Toxicities*: These increase your body's load of heavy metals and solvents/chemicals, affecting your immune system (Crinnion 2003).

17. *Hormones*: High or low levels of hormones, especially changes to the adrenals, affect cervical squamous cells (clinical observation).

18. *Age of First Intercourse*: The younger the age of first intercourse, the higher the risk of cervical dysplasia, as cervical cells are not well developed until the age of 20 (Reich 2006).

19. *Multiple Partners*: Exposes you to more strains and repeat strains of HPV (Reich 2006).

20. *Lack of Support*: Not honoring your path and body's wishes for health leads to disease (Crinnion 2005).

As you can see from this long list that there are indeed many causes which makes your cervix susceptible to the action of HPV. The art of medicine is to work with your physician to identify what area you need to improve in. For example, you may not have the risk factor of having had multiple partners, but perhaps you live in a very polluted city. I encourage you to read the following chapters to gain a better understanding of each of these risk factors, and how they may be affecting your health. I call your risk factor your "*Obstacle to Cure*."

Take Home Message from this Chapter

1. *I have to identify my Obstacle to Cure, because if I don't, the HPV virus will most likely become active on my cervix, leading to pre-cancerous or cancerous lesions.*

Chapter Two

Environmental Toxins

Environmental toxins (i.e., solvents/heavy metals) can create changes to cervical cells in two primary ways: 1) by reducing your antioxidant/nutrient load; and 2) by inducing genetic changes to cell DNA.

Everyday, we are all exposed to toxins. Below is a list of common sources of exposure compiled by my instructor in environmental medicine, Dr. Walter Crinnion, NMD, from lectures in medical school at Southwest College of Naturopathic Medicine in Tempe, Arizona, from 2003 to 2005:

1. **Foods:** If not organic, they tend to be laden with heavy metals, pesticides and herbicides.
2. **Genetically Altered Foods:** Unrecognizable by our bodies.
3. **Cleaning Products**
4. **Odors:** Scented candles, air fresheners and perfumes are made to smell with solvents unless otherwise stated.
5. **Auto Shops:** Solvents and heavy metals.
6. **Auto Exhaust:** Mercury in diesel exhaust can damage the mitochondria of cells, which normally produces our energy (when healthy and mercury-free).
7. **Homes:** Formaldehyde is common, especially in carpets.
8. **Chlorine:** Found in non-filtered water.

9. *Phalates*: Found in some plastics; acts as an estrogen, pushing cancer pathways.
10. *Farmed Salmon*: High in mercury.
11. *Aluminum*: High levels in processed foods and cooking utensils/pans.
12. *Pesticides*: If you spray your lawn, you are being exposed to organochlorines and organophosphates, which are linked to cancer.
13. *Trans Fats/Hydrogenated Oils*: Reduce mitochondrial activity and cell permeability, decreasing cell-to-cell communication.
14. *Tobacco Smoke*: Chemicals in the smoke lead to increased toxin load in cells and decreasing vitamin levels (especially vitamin C).
15. *Mold*: Hard on the immune system, commonly found in older homes/homes damaged by water.
16. *Vaccines*: Mercury is still used as preservative by some companies.
17. *Food Additives*: Such as colorings and preservatives.

General symptoms of toxicities include:

Fatigue
Headaches
Hearing loss
Dizziness
Ringing in ears
Pain (often body-wide)
Arthritis
Degenerative joints
Restless legs
Insomnia
Neurological disorders
Decreased memory
Decreased speech
Weakness
Hormonal changes

Some women will retain more toxins than others. Why is this?

1. *Genetic Differences:* Everyone has different composition of enzyme pathways that help them to detox. Alterations in these biochemical pathways may change the way you break down toxins such as heavy metals or solvents. If you have deficiencies, for example, of these enzymes you will have difficulty breaking down and eliminating toxins. The toxins will then be stored in your tissues as opposed to eliminated.

2. *Trace Mineral/Vitamin Deficiencies:* Either you are not consuming enough vitamins/minerals or not absorbing them properly, which makes levels low. Your body needs a lot of magnesium, trace minerals, B vitamins and vitamin C to process toxins. If it can't process toxins, then the toxin levels build, thereby contributing to the risk of cancer.

3. *High-Sugar/Low-Protein Diets:* Shown clinically to induce cancer and block detox pathways (Kato 1962).

4. *High Stress/Trauma/Emotional Trauma:* All of these situations use up a lot of vitamins and minerals to help you build stress-response hormones while robbing your detox pathways of those same essential nutrients.

5. *Heavy Metals:* Most heavy metals have a long life in your body (ironically called a "half-life") before they are processed out. Mercury fillings, for example, have a half-life of 30 years, meaning in 30 years, half of the original amount will still be in your body.

6. *Increasing Exposure:* A woman living in a toxic city with lots of air pollution puts herself at a higher risk than a woman living in a smaller town or in a rural area where less air pollution exists.

When your body comes into contact with a toxin (called a xenobiotic), it is absorbed through your gut, skin or lungs. Once it is in your body, it is detoxed in two steps called **Phase I** and **Phase II** (before it can be eliminated):

Phase I: This involves systems called cytochrome P450 or glutathione that are highly concentrated in your liver. Cytochrome P450 is composed of groupings of enzymes (i.e., 1A1, 3A are common names for the enzyme groupings), while glutathione is composed primarily of amino acids and vitamin C. Both the cytochrome and glutathione systems are used by your body to initiate the process of breaking down anything your body views as a toxin, including medications. I usually use the analogy of a Ms. Pac-Man game to explain this process: on the screen you see the tiny dots that Ms. Pac-Man has to digest. Those dots are created by **Phase I** enzymes.

Common *Phase I* groupings and the products they break down into Ms. Pac-Man's dots are:

1. *1A and 1B*: Smoke, exhaust
2. *2B*: Medications, such as barbiturates
3. *2E*: Ethanol
4. *3A*: Glucocorticoids, pregnenolone, DHEA, St. John's Wort
5. *1A2*: Common antibiotics
6. *2C*: Antibiotics, anti-depressant medications
7. *3A*: Antibiotics, anti-fungals, grapefruit juice
8. *2E*: Solvents, alcohols
9. *3A4*: Cortisol, estrogen, organophosphates
10. *Glutathione*: Most toxins, especially mercury

Phase II: Going back to the Ms. Pac-Man analogy, imagine those dots in your mind. Ms. Pac-Man is chomping them down. This is *Phase II* (the chomping of dots). Antioxidants are Ms. Pac-Man. Antioxidants bind to the pieces and then help to get them excreted through skin, feces, urine or exhalation (Crinnion 2003). I see a lot of patients as having deficiencies in this part of the detox cycle, which leads to symptoms in a range of conditions not limited to cervical dysplasia, but may include MS, ALS, Parkinson's, osteoarthritis and fibromyalgia, to name a few.

The best treatment of toxins is to avoid them as much as possible. But if you cannot avoid them (i.e., you live in a large polluted city like Phoenix, Arizona), then I recommend you learn to build detoxification into your lifestyle. That being said, one place I like to start with patients who have multiple symptoms (i.e., they have fibromyalgia with cervical dysplasia) is testing their genetic predispositions toward having low *Phase I* or *Phase II* systems. I can also test their inflammatory markers and antioxidant capacity. I use a company called Genova Diagnostics to do these tests.

Genova gives me the ability to get even more specific with women who have a very stubborn history of abnormal pap smears: I can test the level of their mitochondrial function. Mitochondria are called the "powerhouses" of cells, meaning they harness energy from the foods we eat. However, and unfortunately, they are very sensitive to environmental toxins, such as mercury or solvents. (Did you know diesel exhaust is one of the worst sources of mercury and, because of this causes extreme damage to the mitochondria when you breathe it in? Crinnion 2012).

If I feel a patient needs these tests, I will run them before we implement any further treatment regimes. If your body holds onto environmental toxins and if you have a deficiency in one of the pathways thus discussed (cytochrome, glutathione, antioxidant load, for example), then you will have a difficult time reversing the cycle of abnormal pap smears. I guarantee it. And, if you have difficulty with these pathways, your body's levels of key vitamins and minerals will be lower than normal, as your body will be using what it can to keep these processes working.

Inflammation is another very interesting subject. Patients ask me all the time, "Well, isn't inflammation good because it means my immune system is working?" Yes, it does mean it is working, but it may mean it is working too well or too much in the wrong direction. I will refer to Dr. Crinnion's (2012) work once again for this discussion:

> Communication in the immune system occurs by chemical messengers that are typically referred to as cytokines or lymphokines. Included in these chemicals are interferon-gamma, tumor necrosis factor-alpha, a number of interleukins, and a host of other compounds. T-helper cells (Th cells) are also important chemical messengers, functioning to activate or direct other immune cells.

> Th cells are a sub-group of lymphocytes that play an important role in the adaptive immune system... When Th cells proliferate they develop into (1) effector Th cells, (2) memory Th cells, or (3) regulatory Th cells. Effector Th cells subsequently differentiate into two major subtypes known as Type 1 and Type 2 helper T cells (Th1 and Th2 respectively)... Th1 cells... are involved with maximizing the killing efficacy of macrophages, the proliferation of cytotoxic CD+8 T cells, and the production of opsonizing antibodies. Because of this, Th1 cells play a critical role in fighting viral and bacterial pathogens... Th2 cells produce higher levels of interleukin-4 and 5... Th2 over-expression is involved with the promotion of type 1 hypersensitivity... type 2 hypersensitivity (cytotoxic hypersensitivity e.g. "autoimmune conditions"... Th1/Th2 imbalances have been proposed to play a role in immunotoxicity—adverse effects on the functioning of the immune system resulting from exposure to chemical substances.

In very basic terms, environmental toxins push the Th2 pathway relative to the Th1 pathway, and this leads to an inflammatory cascade and autoimmunity. That means your immune system cannot handle or deal with the effects of HPV as well as it could if you did not have toxins in your body.

If I am concerned this is the situation for a patient, we will do the Genova testing and implement supportive supplements or herbs that will support the body to heal. For all patients who want to build detoxification into their everyday routine, I recommend the following:

1. *Avoid sugar*, especially processed sugar, as it suppresses your immune system and causes inflammation.
2. *Avoid foods that are toxic* because of chemicals used to grow them. You can find lists of the most toxic foods on the Environmental Watch Group's home page.
3. *Buy organic foods* whenever possible.
4. *Do not use synthetic cleaning products*, purchase natural ones or make your own.
5. *Do not spray weed-killers* on your lawn. In fact, most people spray to kill weeds like dandelion, which is actually good for your liver!
6. *Purify your body of toxic emotions.* Learn to reduce and let go of anger and resentments.
7. *Get an air purifier* for your home if you live in a new home or if you live in a large city.
8. *Exercise.*
9. *Get lots of sleep*; most people need at least 9 hours per night.
10. *Do not over-work.* (I need to take my own advice here!).
11. *Only listen to music, watch television or movies that are in harmony with your heart.*
12. *Honor yourself*; live and speak your truth, and maintain personal boundaries that are healthy.
13. *Juice fruits and veggies.* This is a great way to get essential nutrients to be absorbed easily by your gut.
14. *Do an infrared sauna daily* for 20 minutes or a few times a week for up to an hour (see below).

15. *Body brush* (see page 11).
16. *Do castor oil packs* over your liver (see page 11).
17. *Consider colonics* if you are really toxic or exposed to toxins regularly (colonics prevent re-absorption of toxic hormones and heavy metals/solvents).
18. *Use the following supplements: Fiber, whey protein, probiotics, vitamin C, B-complex vitamins, and eat good sources of protein* (see Appendix C for a listing of supplements I prescribe).
19. *Vitamin I.V. drips* (see page 11).
20. *Use my multivitamin* because it is awesome! I formulated it for maximum absorption. See my website for details, *howdoitreatnaturally.com* for all Mother Nature's Remedy products (my line).

Of all the treatments listed above, my favorite is the *infrared sauna*. I cannot say enough good things about it. I've had patients who have tried all the latest and greatest supplements, detox plans, fasting, etc., but nothing actually creates change like a good sauna. The wavelength of the infrared causes toxins to be released from cells thereby reducing toxic body load (Kihara et al. 2002).

I recommend patients purchase a FIR Infrared Sauna, which is portable, foldable and looks like a little spaceship, but works well and is affordable. You can purchase one online at *amazon.com* for around $200.

I can tell you numerous stories of patients who, when using the infrared for the first time, noticed either a heavy metal taste in their mouth, got body aches, or had a dramatic decrease in symptoms. These are all signs that toxins are moving.

If you do a sauna and have extreme symptoms, please find a Naturopathic Physician in your area who provides *I.V. drips of vitamin C*. These I.V.s are also laden with magnesium, trace minerals, B vitamins, selenium, zinc and usually extra B-12, which will help your body process all the toxins. For a listing of Naturopathic Physicians in your area, contact your State Naturopathic Association or try the American Association of Naturopathic Physicians at *aanp.org*.

I have patients start with 20 minutes of the sauna either daily or several days a week, depending on their overall health and symptom level. If you have a lot of symptoms related to toxicities, start slower and with shorter time spans. I do not recommend patients sauna more than 30 minutes at a time, as it can feel very depleting, especially if you do a steam sauna (which is not as effective as the infrared in getting out toxins).

Body brushing is a technique that mobilizes your lymphatic cells. Lymph cells move with motion either from exercise or massage. You can purchase a body brush online or from a health food store. Use it very lightly along your skin. Brush from your fingertips to your armpits, from your inner and outer legs upwards, and move everything lightly (you do not have to brush hard to get movement of lymphatics), moving in circular motions towards your heart and liver. This will help move toxins stored in lymphatic tissue to your liver for processing.

Castor oil packs are equally as good at moving lymph and debris out of your liver. Castor oil is commonly sold with a wool cloth, but I have not found this necessary to use (please see my website for the castor oil I use). It is easier to rub a bit of the oil over your liver (which is on the right side of your body, below your ribs), cover with a thin cloth, then apply a hot water bottle to the area and rest for 10-15 minutes. **DO NOT USE A HEATING PAD.** There is something about a heating pad that does not work nearly as well as a hot water bottle.

You may do this treatment daily or a few times a week. It is the most affordable and effective way to boost your liver. The castor oil will absorb through your skin with heat and will then start to move lymphatics. Castor oil is called a "lymphagogue" for its ability to move lymph. Your lymphatics carry a lot of white blood cell debris to your liver for processing.

Case Study: Environmental Toxicity

A patient presented to my office complaining of a history of repeat abnormal pap smears, despite treatment via both LEEP and cryotherapy. She was 44-years-old, still menstruating, and did not have HPV. In fact, she had never had an infection of HPV and had the same sexual partner (her husband) since she was 18 years of age.

She had multiple complaints in addition to cervical dysplasia: fibromyalgia, insomnia, extreme fatigue, frequent headaches and depression. She had experienced most of these symptoms since she was in her early-20s. Upon further questioning, I learned that she had moved to an area of Arizona that was built over what had been a toxic dump, and that their water was laden with solvents as well as heavy metals, such as arsenic. Her symptoms had started within a year of moving to that location.

I reasoned that most of her symptoms might have been related to the exposure to the toxins. We began the following treatment protocol:

Infrared sauna (FIR Infrared) daily for 20 minutes
Body brushing
Castor oil packs over liver
Appropriate supplement support
Increase in antioxidant-rich foods (richly colored foods, like berries)
Vitamin I.V. drips (see page xx)

She responded rapidly to the treatment and had the most benefit from the vitamin I.V. drips. The first symptom that resolved was the body-wide pain. We continued the treatments (she saw me only once a month for an I.V. and did the rest of the treatments on her own), and, after six months, she had a follow-up pap smear.

Her pap was normal for the first time since she was 23.

Take Home Messages from this Chapter

1. *We are all exposed to toxins.*
2. *Supportive supplements/foods/vitamins/minerals are key to healing my cervix.*
3. *Infrared saunas work.*
4. *I need to be consistent with my detox plan.*
5. *Consider Genova Diagnostics testing.*

Chapter Three

Vaccines Against HPV

P atients often ask me my thoughts on the HPV vaccine.

There are 80 (yes, eighty) known strains of HPV, 20 (yes, twenty) of which are linked to cancer. Of the twenty, the vaccine is composed of two strains: strains 16 and 18. That means that 18 of the 20 "cancer-causing strains" you would not be vaccinated for.

I have had patients who had the HPV vaccine and their pap smears were normal, but upon visual inspection of their cervix during the pap exam, I was concerned by what I saw: the appearance was the same as for a woman with an abnormal result. I've also had patients who had the vaccine, but still got an abnormal pap. And, women who did not even have HPV who got an abnormal pap (see *Figure 1*).

Studies are equally conflicting and confusing on this subject. The Lancet published online that "vaccines against cervical dysplasia are highly effective", since the HPV strains 16 and 18 cause 70% of cervical cancers, and cervical cancer is the "second most common type of cancer for women worldwide" (Medscape.com). However, a 4-year, long-term trial found that the vaccines do not decrease the risk of strain 16 and 18 associated cancers (Lehtinen et al. 2012). This was also published in the Lancet Oncology in 2012.

What I will tell you is this: When I do a pap, I am looking at the cervical cells and I take a sample of the cells from that squamous-columnar junction. I see changes on the cervix that look exactly like the changes in the cervixes of women without the vaccine, so something is happening regardless; I worry our current lab testing may be missing something because of the activity of the vaccines.

Male patients want the HPV vaccine, thinking that it would prevent their partners from getting the virus. They also want to be screened for HPV. However, vaccinating men will not stop transmission of a virus; it would only stop symptoms. There is not a consistently good test to identify whether or not men have HPV. Supposedly, an anal swab will identify the virus, but I have ordered this test and it has always come back negative on patients who do have HPV-causing genital warts, which had been previously diagnosed via culture of the lesion.

Recent reports and clinical trials are showing that men can get cancer from HPV. In fact, the rates are higher than I had thought: a staggering 26,000 new cases are diagnosed annually (8,000 in men; Xiocheng Wu et al. 2012). With this in mind, I would like to see laboratory testing to screen men for HPV. My patients tell me their new partners went to get tested for sexually transmitted diseases, were told they are "clean" and had sex without protection. When we re-did their pap smear or did their pap for the first time they now have HPV (or a new strain) showing up. This confirms that the laboratory testing is not conclusive. We need a test for men!

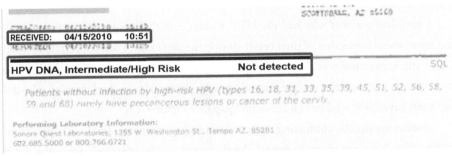

Figure 1: *Patient who does **not** have HPV but, as you will see in the following Figures, still has an abnormal pap.*

*Figure 2. Same patient from **Figure 1** with ASGUS in 2010.*

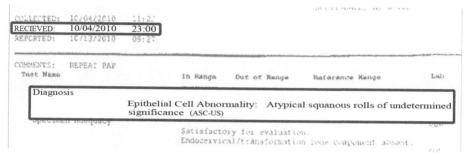

Figure 3. *Patient's re-pap late 2010. Still ASGUS.*
We began treatment a month after this pap was done.

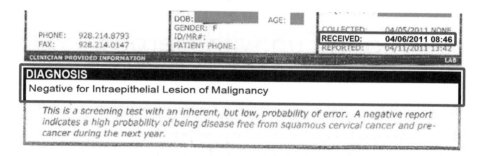

Figure 4. *Approximately four months after **Gowey Protocol®** treatment, normal tissues!*

Take Home Messages from this Chapter

1. *Whether or not I use the vaccine for HPV is personal choice.*
2. *The HPV vaccine may or may not protect me from abnormal pap smear results, as the vaccine is 2 strains of the virus and there are 20 that currently contribute to problems to cervical cells.*
3. *People who have had the vaccine or who have not had HPV may still have an abnormal pap smear result.*
4. *Men can get cancer from HPV, but they probably have obstacles to cure allowing the virus to be active.*

Chapter Four

The Risk New Partners Present and Fun with Herpes

had a patient who had quickly responded to my protocol. Then, months later, her well-woman exam showed the return of the abnormality in her pap. She had been with the same sexual partner the entire time, so what could have happened?

My instincts told me she had acquired a new strain of HPV, a more aggressive one that was causing the new presentation. She had always had ASGUS show in her pap smears, but now she was LSIL. We explored all the possibilities. She had the same partner, but she did not know if he had been with another partner. They used condoms, but could the virus spread despite the condoms? Widespread information on the Internet will tell you that condoms do not lower HPV transmission, but clinical trials disagree. Studies show that condoms do indeed lower HPV transmission (Epstein 2005). We have to remember that HPV, like many viruses, can easily be transmitted via fluid contact. Foreplay, oral and anal sex are possible modes of transmission. Just because you are not having actual intercourse that involves male-female penetration does not make you immune to getting HPV. If you are really worried about HPV, it is always advisable to use a condom, especially with new partners. But, if contracting HPV is unavoidable, remember not to beat yourself up over it. Time and again, I have seen patients living with HPV, with no signs of pre-cancerous lesions.

Studies have also shown that if you already have one strain of HPV, the possibility of acquiring another is much easier and higher. In fact, your risk factor of contracting a new strain is referred to as "high" in the literature (Dennis et al. 2008).

Most women obtain HPV after their first sexual encounter (Dennis et al. 2008). These women also tend to have multiple strains. Longitudinal studies have shown recurrent abnormal pap smears are not necessarily from new or current strains, as detection of multiple strains is common (Dennis et al. 2008). According to work done by Reich (2005), an early age at first intercourse is considered a high risk factor for developing cervical cancer:

...numerous retrospective analyses consider early first intercourse a probable risk factor for later development of cervical carcinoma.

The reason? The area of the cervix susceptible to HPV (at the junction of the two cell types) is not yet developed in younger women. This is especially true for women ages up to 16. This area of cells is termed "the cervical transformation zone" and, at this early age, a lot of the cells are not yet matured. This information also indicates there is no secondary immune response at this early age to HPV.

In patients with repeat abnormal pap smears, I would screen for other STDs (sexually transmitted diseases). Patients with diseases, such as bacterial vaginosis or Chlamydia, commonly have abnormal pap smears:

Lifestyle, Chlamydia, trachomotis infection, bacterial vaginosis, HIV all increase the tendency to have abnormal paps from HPV. (Zbroch et al. 2004)

All of my patients worry about co-infection with other viruses. Herpes is the most common virus I get asked about. There are two strains of herpes: HSV I and HSV II. HSV I used to be thought of as a "kissing disease", while HSV II was thought to cause problems on genitalia. Now, there is no real distinction between the two; and herpes manifestations of either strain can be found on almost any body part. In fact, there is now an insurance diagnostic code for almost any body part. I learned this while doing a clinical trial in 2011, whereby I compared the **Gowey Protocol® Gel** (see *Chapter 13*) to placebo on 32 patients (double-blind, placebo controlled study—see Appendix A for results). Patients were presenting to the study with herpes manifestations anywhere from their buttocks to their necks. Most were on the lips (known affectionately as a "cold sore"). Cold sores and genital breakouts of herpes can be extremely painful, itchy or tingly, and can last for weeks. The **Gowey Protocol®** **Gel**, however, reduced symptoms dramatically within two days relative to placebo and patients experienced an instant reduction in pain with the first application of the **Gel**. It is an amazing plant that I'm working with.

I tell all my patients that herpes is nothing to fear. Almost everyone has it, with estimates from 50-90% of the global population, depending on socioeconomic area or country. Some people get breakouts of it and some do not; the ones who do tend to have a lot of stress. Stress lowers vitamin levels and suppresses your immune system, which then allows the virus to become active and cause symptoms. For herpes, follow the suggestions I pose with regards to immune/vitamin support (see *Chapters 5 and 7*), use my **Gel** if you get a breakout, and do not worry about it beyond that. This is not something to be ashamed of; you can heal your body from herpes just as you can from HPV. Do not give the virus any more energy than what it deserves.

Case Study: Herpes Outbreak

A young woman presented to my office with a sudden, acute outbreak of herpes. This was her first experience with it and she had recently had her blood levels checked showing she did have HSV I (the herpes strain thought to only cause cold sores). She had several new lesions on her external labia (the layers of skin along your clitoris) causing her extreme pain.

Without thinking, I found myself reaching for the **Gowey Protocol®** **Gel**, applying the **Gel** to each lesion. I suddenly felt like I was in slow motion; as if time had stopped and I was an observer watching myself apply the **Gel** to her lesions. Her boyfriend and I stared in amazement at how she reacted to the **Gel**. Almost immediately, she stopped crying. She calmed down and she breathed a sigh of relief. She said that the pain stopped as soon as I started to apply the **Gel**.

Following up with her, she said the lesions had crusted over within 48 hours of that initial application, which is a sign of healing. I had given her some of the **Gel** to continue using every hour or two. She has not had symptoms of herpes since this outbreak, as she applies the **Gel** as soon as she may feel any tingling or sensations that she is getting an outbreak.

Take Home Messages from this Chapter

1. *Herpes is nothing to be ashamed of.*
2. *Most people in the world have herpes.*
3. *My partner may carry more than one strain of HPV, and may carry other viruses such as herpes (or HIV).*
4. *I can successfully treat the symptoms of herpes.*

Chapter Five

Nutrition

Nutrition is key when treating any condition, but especially cervical dysplasia. Without good nutrition and vitamin levels, your body's immune system will not be able to prevent HPV from taking hold and you will be more susceptible to developing cancerous cells. I start with patients by taking a thorough investigation into their diets. We begin by discussing what foods to avoid and why:

1. **Food Sensitivities:** We all have food sensitivities, the level of which is different for everyone. Some people have symptoms from foods they are sensitive to, and some do not. Symptoms can range from rashes to mood swings. Why the difference? Partly genetics, partly the health of the food you are eating (eating organic is always better), partly stress, and partly from the ways foods combine when you eat them. The biggest problems arise when a patient is under a lot of stress. Stress increases the hormone cortisol, which helps your body maintain its basic functions (such as blood sugar levels) while you are going through the stress. Unfortunately, the elevation in cortisol suppresses an immune cell called Secretory IgA, which normally creates a mucosal membrane on your intestinal tract. This lining both protects your gut and helps you absorb nutrients. Under stress, the cortisol blocks the action of the Secretory IgA, the mucosal membrane does not get built, and your absorption of nutrients

changes. Proteins that you could normally digest escape into the blood stream whole causing diseases such as Irritable Bowel Syndrome.

2. *Reducing Inflammatory Reactions:* Food sensitivities also cause inflammation. This inflammatory reaction can cause problems such as arthritis, eczema, ear infections (especially in children), chronic cold/flu, depression, diarrhea, anxiety, autoimmune diseases, and of course, cervical dysplasia. This inflammatory reaction is called a "delayed sensitivity reaction", meaning it can take time (hours to days) before symptoms result. There are four different types of immune cells responsible for this reaction, called IgG's, and they are numbered 1-4. Subtype 1 tends to be a reaction that shows up within an hour or two (meaning, the IgG binds to the proteins in the food your body views as foreign and causes symptoms), while IgG subtype 4 reactions take days to show symptoms. This can make identifying the foods you are truly sensitive to difficult, especially if you only eat them every few days. The most common foods I see causing this include eggs, dairy products, wheat products and beans. I recommend patients either do what is called an elimination diet, which involves removing one food at a time for at least 9-14 days to watch for symptom changes (it can take that long for the IgG levels to lower), or doing my favorite food sensitivity panel by Immunolabs. This company has a fantastic test of 154 of the most common foods and ranks them in subtypes 1-4. Please ask your health care provider about this test if you would like to do it, or contact me to have it ordered.

3. *Wheat:* I have started to see more and more people, especially babies, sensitive to wheat and wheat products. I've learned that the companies who provide seeds to farmers are now changing the way the grains are genetically modified to be "immune" to chemicals, such as 2,4-D, which is a known carcinogen. I am recommending to my patients that they go gluten-free or avoid wheat.

4. *Dairy:* I think the problem we have with dairy products is: 1) The dairy protein make-up is nothing like our own (mother's milk); and 2) Cow's milk is commonly full of hormones and antibiotics used in raising the animals. I recommend patients who are sensitive to dairy try goat-milk products or go organic.

5. *Soy:* Extracts from soy (isoflavones) have been demonstrated to increase the risk of developing CIN I. For example, the isoflavone (a compound in soy) enterodiol has been associated with an increased CIN I risk. However, I

have only seen this clinically to be the case if you are eating high amounts of foods with this constituent. Eating them occasionally, I have not seen to be a problem unless you have a specifically identified food sensitivity reaction to soy (Hernandez 2004).

6. *Sugar:* I should have a website called *sugarispoison.com* (sorry, processed sugar industry, but you are not helping us prevent cancer). Because, while I, like any other human being, likes her chocolate cake now and again, sugar is really bad for you, plain and simple. Processed sugars usurp your body of nutrients, as they take more energy and resources to get energy from these sugars than they contribute. We also learned in Naturopathic school that your immune system is suppressed for 4-6 hours upon consumption of only one teaspoon of simple, white (processed) sugar. I recommend that, if you have a sweet tooth, you try cooking or sweetening with Stevia or other all-natural sweeteners.

7. *Supplement Absorption:* Most supplements, I hate to say, do not absorb well. Really do your homework before purchasing any brand of supplements, stick to brands in health food stores, or consider brands I have listed in the Appendix. I have also worked very hard to bring to you supplements and various herbal formulations that are designed for maximum absorption and efficacy (for more information, go to my website, *howdoitreatnaturally.com*). This work has been based on over 15 years of experience in the supplement and natural foods industry (I got my start in my early-20s as a Buyer for Whole Foods Market).

8. *Alcohol Use:* Depletes key vitamins such as B-12 and magnesium.

You can heal your gut by avoiding foods you are sensitive to, managing your stress levels (i.e., via good sleep or exercise), taking probiotics, or use formulas designed for repairing your gut lining (Integrative Therapeutics has a good one called Permeability Factors but I am also working on one which I hope to have out in 2013 or 2014).

Case after case has shown how low levels of nutrients increases the risk of cervical dysplasia (and cervical cancer), such as:

Low vitamins A, C, Bs (Liv et al. 1993)
Low B-12 (Kwanbunjan et al. 2006)
Low beta carotene, lycopene, zeaxanthin, lutein, retinol (Cho et al. 2009)

Low vitamin E (Cho et al. 2009)
50% higher risk with low serum concentration of tocopherols and reduced intake of dark green leafy greens or deep yellow veggies (Tomita et al. 2010)
Lower folate levels (Flatley et al. 2009)
Low antioxidant levels increase free radical damage on the cervix (Basu 2005)
Low vitamin C increases free radical damage (Lee et al. 2005)
Low trace minerals such as selenium and zinc (Kim et al. 2003)
Too high of mineral levels such as heavy metals (Kim et al. 2003)

I found that most articles and studies linked low antioxidant levels and reduced detoxifying enzyme systems (see *Chapter 2*) to cervical dysplasia and cancer. One study in particular looked at manganese superoxide dismutase (SOD), which is the primary antioxidant enzyme/mineral combination inside of the mitochondria of every cell in your body. The study found that low SOD levels are not necessarily associated with increased cervical dysplasia and cancer, but SOD without the mineral manganese are. Additionally, low antioxidants that normally work with or are associated with SOD (such as lycopene, zexanthin, lutein, and vitamin E) show an increased risk in cervical dysplasia (Tong et al. 2009). Manganese SOD is the primary antioxidant enzyme in mitochondria, which are key to protecting cells from oxidative stress and is needed for all enzymatic activities carried out by the mitochondria.

Another study found antioxidant levels to be low in CIN patients and even lower in patients with cervical cancer. This same study looked at the effects of "lipid peroxidation" on CIN level, finding a positive correlation. Lipid peroxidation comes from the effects of eating trans fats, fried foods or hydrogenated oils and having low antioxidant levels. Your body cannot recognize or convert these fats into useable forms for your cells, and fats are needed for the building of every cell membrane in your body (Kim et al. 2003).

I am seeing more and more the importance of minerals such as magnesium for overall health. I learned in medical school that low magnesium is the most common mineral deficiency in the United States, in part due to the low levels of foods consumed that has magnesium (high in leafy greens), but also because of low levels in soil. I would argue that minerals in general, including trace minerals, are low for almost everyone. If someone presents to me with high blood pressure, which is extremely common, I always consider increasing the patient's magnesium/trace mineral levels. Magnesium is needed to dilate blood vessels and relax muscles, while calcium contracts. Patients tend to be higher in calcium relative to magnesium, which can and does result in high blood pressure. It can also result in abnormal changes in your cervix.

Common causes of low magnesium/low trace mineral levels include:

Alcohol consumption (Tolstrup et al. 2006)
Hormonal disorders such as hypothyroid/hyperthyroidism or adrenal fatigue
Processed sugar in diet
Low leafy green consumption
Use of medications, such as diuretics
Liver diseases
Stress
Acidic extracellular fluids

I treat mineral levels via vitamin I.V. drips that have vitamin C, B complex, magnesium, manganese, zinc, selenium, chromium, calcium, and extra B12. I also recommend to patients they use liquid or powder mineral supplements (or juice their fruits and veggies), as absorption tends to be better relative to tableted products.

An increase in body acidity has also been linked to cancer. Your body's blood pH is kept at 7.4. Your blood cannot stray from the pH of 7.4; if it deviates from 7.4 even a little, death will result. Your body works hard at keeping your blood pH at 7.4, and uses minerals to do so. If your pH starts to drop below 7.4 (acidic) your body will mobilize calcium, sodium and potassium from bone to neutralize the blood pH back to 7.4. Foods that your body views as "acidic" include (Aihara 1986):

Sugar (i.e., sugary snacks/deserts/soda)
Animal Proteins/Proteins
Refined Foods (processed foods)
Chemical Additives (to foods)
Grains
Beans (because of the high protein content)
Alcohol (beer)

If you consume high amounts of these types of foods, you are keeping your body more acidic and, therefore, your bones will lose minerals like calcium to maintain the right blood pH.

Conversely, there are foods that create more of an alkaline body environment. These include:

Fruits
Vegetables
Miso/Soy Products
Wine
Rice

You can test to see if you are getting the right balance of acid to alkaline by testing the pH of your urine. I recommend you take the pH test a few times a day. You can order pH strips online, or local pharmacies may carry them. Ideally, your urine pH should be around 6-7. If it is higher, you are alkaline (which is fine), but if it's lower than 6, you are too acidic and need to increase your intake of vegetables. As you adjust your diet, you will see changes reflected in your urine pH. I challenge you to drink a soda and then test your pH for the next few hours and days. You will be amazed at the results.

Case Study: Go Nutrition!

I had a patient who only used the *Gowey Protocol® Gel* and did vitamin I.V. drips every two weeks to treat her HPV. For her, this was enough. She saw a change for the better in her pap results within three months. Overall, she was the healthiest patient I had worked with; she was not on any birth control, was very conscientious about her diet, did regular exercise and cleanses. She cleansed by juice fasting every few months.

If you are going to do a type of cleanse that involves fasting, I do not recommend not eating, as there are too many environmental toxins (see Chapter 2) that begin to circulate out of fat cells as soon as you start to decrease your caloric intake. If you do juices while fasting or cleansing, you will be giving your body antioxidant support (remember Ms. Pac-Man?) to bind to the toxins and help remove them from your body. Cleansing would also be a good time to add something like the infrared sauna (see *Chapter 2*).

This patient welcomed my sharing the results of her paps with you (*Figures 5 and 6*). Notice the time period it took her to get better, and she has not had an abnormal pap since we worked together.

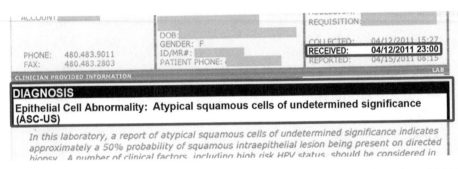

Figure 5. Pap prior to starting treatment of vitamin I.V. drips (ASGUS) as of April 2011.

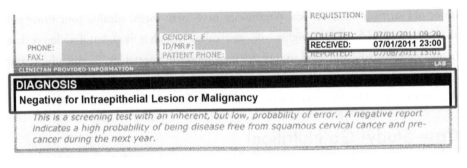

Figure 6. Pap results less than three months later—normal tissues.

Take Home Messages from this Chapter

1. *Nutrition is key to improving the outcomes from an abnormal pap.*
2. *Processed sugars are not good for me.*
3. *Antioxidants are key to cervical health.*

Chapter Six

Genetic Variability

have had patients with abnormal paps who do not have HPV. *The British Journal of Cancer* published a study in 2010 demonstrating that 10% of women with abnormal paps do not have HPV (Mesher et al. 2010). It would be difficult to fully ascertain the degree to which this is true; up until recently, most practitioners ran the pap test without typing for HPV, or ordered the HPV test only if the pap returned abnormal. Therefore, it would truly be impossible to tell just how many women have dysplasia with or without HPV.

The TERC gene has been identified as a marker for abnormal paps in women with HPV (Anderson et al. 2009). Genetic marker CCR2 has been identified in women with cervical dysplasia independent of HPV. According to this study, some women will have abnormal paps no matter what they do to treat themselves. I would not jump to this conclusion independent of a study comparing the **Gowey Protocol®** to a placebo in women who do have the CCR2 gene and women who do not. Until that study is done, I would imagine that any woman who truly believes, and who is truly willing to invest in herself, would be able to prevent the deleterious effects of the CCR2 gene on her body.

Here are some of the thoughts from a patient who was willing to invest in herself:

When I had my first abnormal pap and found out I had HPV, my first thought was, 'I'm not a promiscuous person, how could this happen to me? The first thing I did, which was probably a mistake, was to go online to find out what HPV was. After a little bit of reading, I didn't feel much better. All I got out of it was cancer! But my doctor had assured me that I was going to be fine and that it was going to go away.

Two years and two colposcopies later, I was still having abnormal paps with HPV. I began to get more worried and was trying to figure out what I was doing wrong. After meeting with Dr. Gowey and having true reassurance that she could help me, I finally felt relief. The idea of cancer, after seeing my own mother battle breast cancer, truly frightened me. But, after beginning the Protocol with the combination of vitamin I.V.s and supplements, I really did feel good. The idea of a monthly visit to the doctor seemed invasive but, looking back, it was well worth it. I now feel more educated and more aware of my sexual health. I'm honest with people about my personal experience of being diagnosed with HPV and it has made it so many of my friends feel comfortable talking about their sexual health. As women, we are burdened with the diagnosis of HPV, since men are carriers and cannot be tested for it. HPV is not something to be ashamed of. — L., Phoenix, AZ

I have a patient with MS who was told by his dad (who also has MS) that, because the family history includes MS, there is no way he could get better. I disagreed with his statement; if we were all entirely controlled by our genetics, no one would be alive. I have seen clinically that, if you work to improve your nutrition, limit your exposure to environmental toxins and detox regularly, you can change the way your body responds to genetic alterations. There is a process called "apoptosis" that involves the recognition and destruction of abnormal cells. This apoptosis is improved and increased by antioxidants in color-rich berries (remember the Ms. Pac-Mans).

My friend and colleague, Dr. Jon Kalman, NMD, told me his theory on antioxidants that I found quite interesting: He said that he eats berries by the pound in the summer, and it always takes away sunburns by the next day. Why is it that the earth gives us berries in the summer? Think about it!

Take Home Messages from this Chapter

1. *My individual genetics may be preventing me from getting better.*
2. *I can affect my genetic expression by improving my overall health.*
3. *I can increase the Ms. Pac-Mans in my body with antioxidant-rich foods, such as berries.*

Chapter Seven

The Role of the Immune System

Without a good, healthy, active immune system, your body will struggle to beat HPV at its game. Seresini (et al. 2010) identified anti-HPV18 CD4 T cells, a type of immune cell that usually responds to the presence of a virus and clear the HPV infection. CD4 T cells eliminate the presence of HPV on cervical cells.

In my experience, you have to look at many factors in order to support your immune system:

Vitamin/mineral levels
Potentially low detox pathways
Environmental exposure
Stress levels
Sugar consumption
Food sensitivities
Hormone levels

Hormones, whether they are too high or too low, can have a suppressive affect on your immune system. Think of women who are pregnant; they tend to get colds easily. Their hormones, such as progesterone, are very high and this can impact the immune system in a negative way.

You also need to eliminate foods you are sensitive to; those foods create inflammation, which then can suppress your immune system. If you are someone who gets a cold or the flu frequently, you most likely have food sensitivities. Herbs can help your immune system; I have a formula of immune herbs that I blended just for my dsyplasia patients. It is available on my website.

There are a few treatments I highly recommend for boosting the immune system and, of those, one of my favorites is called "contrast hydrotherapy".

Hydrotherapy is "water therapy", and was popularized in the 1900s by a French priest, Father Sebastian Kneipp, who, while very ill, had run across a water therapy book written by a physician (whom he never named in his book). He tried dozens of these water treatments on himself and remained "rigorous" all the days of his life, which he attributed to the water treatments.

Hydrotherapy applications were a cornerstone of my medical training. I prescribe these treatments for lung infections (i.e., bronchitis), sore throats, chronic diseases, arthritis, and now: cervical dysplasia! I will be coming out with an instructional video in late 2012 showing you how to do home constitutional hydrotherapy.

Hot compresses (a compress is a towel or washcloth) applied to the skin cause blood vessels to dilate. If you then switch the hot compress for a cold application, the vessels initially constrict, but then they dilate again to warm the skin. This creates a "pumping" action, moving blood cells (including immune system cells) to the area you are treating.

The best, most effective treatment I have seen (which I learned in medical school during our hydrotherapy courses, handed down by Dr. Letitia Watrous, ND, of Spokane, WA) is as follows:

1. *Get two cotton towels that extend from your throat to waistline, a wool or fleece blanket, and two basins of water—one hot and one cold.*
2. *Saturate one towel in hot water (not so hot as to burn your skin, just nice and warm), wring it out well so it is not dripping with water, and place from throat to waist (this works best if you are naked). Cover the towel with your wool or fleece blanket to keep you warm (you may cover with other blankets, as well; it is key not to get cold at all during this treatment).*
3. *Rest five minutes.*

4. Take the other towel and dip in the cold water, wring out well, replace the hot towel with the cold one, and then cover again with the wool or fleece blanket(s). Remember to stay warm; do not allow yourself to get chilled.

5. Rest 10 minutes.

6. Check the cold towel with your hand. It should start to feel warm. If not, rest five more minutes. This is a test of your vitality; if you are constitutionally weak, you will not warm this towel well.

7. Repeat the cycle at least two more times for a total of no less than 45 minutes.

If you feel your immune system is struggling with the **Gowey Protocol®**, then I recommend you do these treatments a few days a week.

Case Study: Immune Support

I had a patient who only did alternating hot/cold treatments and took some herbs to boost her immune system. After a few months of treatment, we did a repeat pap smear; her results are in *Figures 7 & 8*.

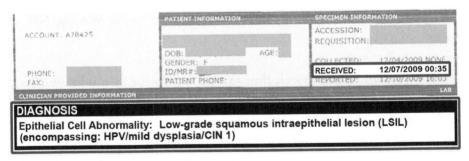

Figure 7. Pre-treatment pap (CIN I).

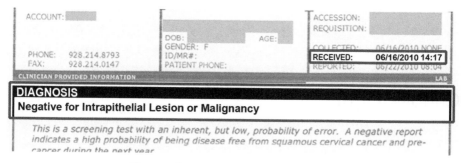

Figure 8. *Post-Protocol pap is normal.*

Take Away Messages from this Chapter

1. *My immune system needs to be healthy to conquer the potential deleterious effects of HPV.*
2. *I can boost my immune system in different ways.*
3. *Alternating hot and cold water treatments to my skin will increase my immune system.*

Chapter Eight

What You Say=
What You Get

have much respect and admiration for people like Joel Osteen. He reaches millions of people weekly through his television and Internet broadcasts, and travels the world with his message of hope and restoration. I can sum up his messages in this quote:

Whatever you feed will grow. — Joel Osteen

Have you ever stopped to think about what you think about, or what you say, to yourself or to others? If you were to write down what you think about and what you say, then write down your life events or current situation, do they match? If you say you are healthy, chances are you will be. If you say you are sick, chances are you will be.

Every week, I listen to the broadcasts done by Joel Osteen (*joelosteen.com*). Lately, he's been talking about how what we say equals what we get. He says, "The first place we must win the victory is in our own minds."

As a person thinks in his/her heart, so he/she will become. — Proverbs 23:7

I often see what patients say as dictating their future. What people say is an extension of their thoughts and, if the Universe is built upon principles within physics,

36

and if thought forms have an energy, then what you think or say would match what comes physically to form.

In my professional opinion, the biggest contributing factor and cause of HPV-induced cervical dysplasia is one's emotional state, one's feelings toward the virus, and one's self-image.

Most women get HPV from their first partner; this is not always the case, but it is common. This oftentimes comes with a feeling of shame. I often hear statements such as:

"I waited to have sex with him until he was committed to me, but he gave me HPV anyway."
"He/she had an affair, and I got it from that new partner."
"He told me he was clean of all disease."
"I had an affair and got it from my new partner."
"I fell in love, but he just used me and gave me HPV."
"He/she left me for another woman/man, but only after he/she gave me HPV."
"I was raped and got it."
"I trusted we were committed and had unprotected sex, and I got it."
"He/she told me they didn't have it but they were wrong/they lied."
"I didn't think that having unprotected sex just once could give it to me."

Do any of these quotes resonate with you? You are not alone and I want you to know you should not feel ashamed. There is nothing to feel shame over—absolutely nothing. This virus is not your fault.

A patient once asked me to ask the virus why it hurts us, causes suffering or cancer. In a meditative state, I asked the virus and the answer I got may surprise you. I felt, deep inside me, the virus' energy, and it was saying that it was just "living out its path", living its lifecycle and following how it was designed to survive, not meaning any ill-intention. It was from this meditation that this book was sprung, as I realized that we are in control of more than what we think. If we truly take our health to heart, and truly work on our wellness, we can get better. That may not be the case in women who have genetic abnormalities that allow the virus to be very active, but even with that said, you do have the power to influence your genetics through diet, healthy hormone levels, detoxing, good nutrient levels, and your mindset.

Please take away the negative association with this virus from your mind. It is more important to use this time of healing to manifest the healthy state you desire for your body, mind and spirit, and take the necessary steps to bring that desired state into reality.

I have a patient who was beginning to incorporate the things I am sharing with you into her lifestyle. She was eating better, cutting back on alcohol consumption, and focusing on good sleep and exercise. However, her paps were not improving. We discussed her mindset; while she was a very, very positive person in her work, she was not as positive in her private life. We discussed positive mantras she could do as well as self-talk, such as: "I am healthy! My cervix is gorgeous! I am happy and doing well! My body deserves health. I deserve health!"

I got an email from her a few weeks later telling me, "I'm going to kick this thing!" It was so powerfully stated that I knew beyond a doubt she would indeed get better. And she did! Within a short time after that emailed declaration, her cervix began to change in appearance, her energy strengthened, her smile deepened, and she became whole; a beautiful woman with a healthy, normal pap result.

What are you allowing your mind to dwell on? Are you focused on your problems? Are you constantly dwelling on negative things? How you view your life makes all the difference in the world, especially for you.

— Joel Osteen (2011)

Pastor Joel Osteen is not the only leader in our society who agrees. Abraham Hicks would tell you that, "worry creates the future you are trying to avoid." Dr. Dossey, MD, has this to add, from his book, Healing Words:

Research in the field of psychosomatic medicine has demonstrated beyond reasonable doubt that disturbances in the mind can cause bodily dysfunction and disease "within an individual" and "between individuals." Studies at Princeton University's Engineering Anomalies Research Laboratory (PEAR Lab) have shown people can influence outcomes of physical events and can mentally convey information to others, even from across the globe. In fact, amazingly, the receiver of that message "gets" that information three DAYS before the event.

Dossey likes to tell the story of the Patron Saint Peregrine. He had cancer and was scheduled for amputation of the leg because of it. The night before the procedure, he prayed fervently that he was healed. During sleep, he had a dream that he was well; in fact, when he awoke, he was. He lived to 80-years-old, dying cancer-free in 1345.

I love a little book written by Doreen Virtue called **Angel Words**, which actually shows the physical frequency of words and phrases. Words that are positive have a higher vibration as compared to words that are negative. If you do not believe me, try this experiment: Say all manner of negative things for one solid day and see how you feel by the end of that day as well as the course of events throughout the day. Then, the next day, say nothing but good things, to yourself, your body, your friends and your family. Smile even if you don't want to and, at the end of that day, see how you feel!

If you are new to prayer, or wonder how to do it, it is quite simple: ASK–THANK–EXPECT. The key is staying in a place of gratitude, accepting your life situations that you cannot change, and always moving forward into greatness.

And it shall come to pass, that before they call, I will answer. — Isaiah 65:24

Your cervix is beautiful, healthy and whole. You are beautiful, healthy and whole. Believe it, see it in your mind, and then live it! Your cervix looks like a nice, pink donut. Visualize it!

Dr. B's treatment plan gave me great strength to overcome not only the "disease", but also the anxiety of conquering the virus while waiting for good results. The power of a good attitude, Dr. B's amazing Gel, and surrounding yourself with positive people just turns this nightmare into peace. The key to this plan is to follow the Protocol and make sure to feed your mind with positive quotes, books, humor, laughter, and fun.
Life is too short. Get rid of the negative energy and only allow the good to creep into your body. It makes a world of difference. — K, Scottsdale, AZ

Case Study: Emotional Health

I've been dealing with HPV for 10 years now, and I've had abnormal pap smears for 10 years. I started seeing Doctor Gowey when I was told that

I would need to have a layer of my cervix burned off to try to re-grow new cells. I was told that this was my best option and getting rid of HPV. Well, after some research, I learned that it isn't a cure and that it can really damage my cervix. I'm only 30-years-old, and having kids is very important to me. I wasn't at all happy with the suggestion that this was the only option. After years of pap smears every three months, and numerous biopsies, I decided to seek other treatment. I began seeing Dr. Gowey, and she had me focus on my diet and vitamins. Over these last 10 years, I've had a lot of toxic friends in my life, which, in turn, created a lot of drama around me, and my health suffered. I was constantly stressed out and getting sick. I was run down and just plain unhappy. I recently got rid of those toxic friends and, along with these vitamins, for the first time in 10 years, I had my first normal pap smear. So, while vitamins, sleep and diet are a very key point in being healthy, I also feel those people you surround yourself with play a key role in that, as well. — J, Flagstaff, AZ

This patient had a most amazing story. She had been working with me for months to improve, but she was sick all the time. It seemed like every time I turned around, she was sick again with a cold or flu. After several months of counseling her on diet changes and immune support, she decided to do treatment on her own for a while.

I did not see her for a year. Yes, I was worried because she was CIN III.

She came to me after one year for a repeat pap. In that time, she had not seen any gynecologists. She was perfectly healthy and had not been sick in months. She had decided to not talk to people in her life that she had decided were "toxic", and it was at that point that she stopped being so sick.

When I inserted the speculum for her pap, I just about fell off my little, rolly stool. Her cervix was absolutely gorgeous. When I had first started to treat her, I had met her post-colposcopy; the cervix was red, irritated and looked like raw hamburger. The **Gowey Protocol® Gel** had healed the hamburger-like appearance, but the dysplasia had still been there when last we met. When we got her new pap results back, they were totally normal! Her pap is below. She did not use the plant **Gel** during this time, only positive affirmations.

I also wanted to share with you her diet diary, which she shared with me at the one-year follow-up visit:

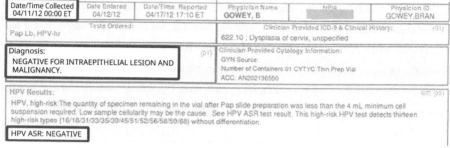

| Date/Time Collected 04/11/12 00:00 ET | Date Entered 04/12/12 | Date/Time Reported 04/17/12 17:10 ET | Physician Name GOWEY, B | NPI# | Physician ID GOWEY,BRAN |

Figure 9. Normal pap after treatment of avoiding "toxic" people in her life.

Food Journal

Friday, 3/9 – Coffee, cereal, water, ham/artichoke sandwich, salad, red wine, almonds

Saturday, 3/10 – Scrambled eggs with salsa, coffee, OJ, water, deer jerky, chicken fajitas, beer, almonds

Sunday, 3/11 – Coffee, Jack in the Box burger and fries, Coke, steak with mushrooms, asparagus, red wine, chocolate pudding, almonds

Monday, 3/12 – Coffee, OJ, Water, hard boiled egg, toast, strawberries, almonds, protein shake, red wine, roasted chicken, salad, mashed potatoes

Tuesday, 3/13 – Coffee, OJ, water, oatmeal with strawberries, deer jerky, almonds, ham sandwich, chips, leftover steak, roasted carrots, red wine

Wednesday, 3/14 – Coffee, OJ, cereal with strawberries, scrambled eggs with cheese and salsa burrito, water, beer, red wine, beef taquitos, beans and rice

Thursday, 3/15 – Water, coffee, egg/ham sandwich, beet salad, almonds, beer, roasted shrimp, broccoli, and asparagus, milk, chocolate pudding with strawberries

Friday, 3/16 – Water, coffee, glazed donut, scrambled eggs with cheese and salsa burrito, OJ, champagne, roasted artichoke, red wine, chocolate pudding

Saturday, 3/17 – Water, coffee, scrambled eggs with cheese and salsa burrito, OJ, chicken fingers, fries, beer

Sunday, 3/18 – Coffee, eggs, toast, bacon, OJ, beer, roasted chicken, mashed potatoes, salad, red wine, magic cookie bar, milk

Monday, 3/19 – Coffee, oatmeal with strawberries, salad with chicken, magic cookie bar, water, deer jerky, spaghetti, red wine, magic cookie bar, milk

Tuesday, 3/20 – *Coffee, blueberry oat bar, almonds, water, deer jerky, cereal, beer, roasted chicken leftovers, mashed taters, steamed broccoli, red wine, milk, magic cookie bar*

Wednesday, 3/21 – *Coffee, blueberry oat bar, protein shake, deer jerky, water, almonds, red wine, salad, chicken with asparagus, pasta*

Thursday, 3/22 – *Coffee, cereal with strawberries, OJ, leftover roasted chicken, mashed potatoes, apple, Triscuits, water, M&M's, (can't remember what I had for dinner)*

Notice she was consuming alcohol and sugar, both foods that I had shared may be linked to abnormal paps. She was still consuming some of these items, so this means they were not her obstacles to cure; the unhealthy relationships were. I bring this up because I want you to take home the message that you may not need to do all the things I recommend. It's good to start with as many of these as you can because, in that time and learning process, you will learn what is your obstacle to cure. Once you learn that, you can either avoid it or deal with it.

Case Study: ASGUS to LSIL

A 55-year-old patient presented to me with a new diagnosis of HPV, which she had gotten for the first time in her life. She had never had an abnormal pap before and was concerned that she now was ASGUS. We increased her nutritional levels, increased her immune support, and I had her insert the **Gowey Protocol® Gel** several times per week. As the owner of a hair salon, she handles solvents and chemicals regularly. I discussed this with her as a possible contributing factor to the ASGUS.

After months of working together, we finally achieved a pap that did not show any dysplasia. She took the results to her OB/GYN's office. There, she was told that because she still had HPV she needed the LEEP. If she did the LEEP, they said, it would cause the HPV to go away. Ladies, this is not true. LEEP does not remove the presence of the virus.

Needless to say, this report from her gynecologist scared her deeply. She became very fearful and, in a few months, her pap came back as ASGUS again. She went back to this office, unbeknownst to me, and had the LEEP done. Unfortunately, this office did not do a colposcopy on her first.

Six months later, she came back to me for her repeat pap. This one was worse, LSIL, and, not only that: her cervix was covered in what appeared to be scar tissue (I often see this post-LEEP or even post-colposcopy). What was so powerful about this visit was not so much that her pap had come back abnormal, but that she knew what had caused it to be worse. These were her exact words:

"I realize now that my thoughts and my emotions are giving me cancer."

So powerful! How many of us have negative thoughts or emotions no matter what your life situation is? And how many of us are giving ourselves abnormal pap smears by our own intention? I know that life has so many hardships and challenges, and that relationships can be very difficult to sort through; I am not putting down anyone's experience. What I am doing is pointing out how very real our emotions are to our bodies, and that we do need to do the work on ourselves if we want to get better.

You may not be able to change anyone else, but you can change you. I remind women that others have their own journey, and that you have yours. No one makes us happy but us! We have to make the conscious choice to be happy and healthy.

My patient's pap that had gone back to LSIL is on the right:

I recently ran across a clinical trial linking our immune and neurological systems (Skaper et al. 2012). In this study, researchers found that immune markers called "proinflammatory cytokines", which are molecules allowing communication between immune cells, signal neurological system cells called "glia" to cross over into the central nervous system. This causes what the researchers called "neuroinflammation" (inflammation of your nervous system). The nervous system inflammation then signals back to your immune system that there is a problem, and the cascade continues. This is what happens on your cervix. Your body literally hears the message from you that something is wrong (perhaps it started with a negative thought), and then this signals

Date/Time Collected 04/06/12 00:00 ET	Date Entered 04/07/12	Date/Time Reported 04/16/12 09:36 ET	Physician Name GOWEY, B	NPI#	Physician ID GOWEY,BRAN
Tests Ordered: Pap Lb, HPV-hr; Physician Read Pap			Clinician Provided ICD-9 & Clinical History: 795.1 ; Abnormal Papanicolaou smear of vagina and vaginal HPV		(01)
Diagnosis: EPITHELIAL CELL ABNORMALITY. LOW-GRADE SQUAMOUS INTRAEPITHELIAL LESION (LSIL); MILD DYSPLASIA IS PRESENT.	(01)	Clinician Provided Cytology Information: GYN Source: Number of Containers:01 CYTYC Thin Prep Vial			
HPV Results: HPV, high-risk:The quantity of specimen remaining in the vial after Pap slide preparation was less than the 4 mL minimum cell suspension required. Low sample cellularity may be the cause. See HPV ASR test result. This high-risk HPV test detects thirteen high-risk types (16/18/31/33/35/39/45/51/52/56/58/59/68) without differentiation.					(02) (03)
HPV ASR: POSITIVE					

Figure 10. LSIL pap.

to your immune system that all is not well, which in turn tells your nervous system the same thing.

As a physician, I firmly believe that you need to be extremely mindful of your thoughts and emotions. Find the support you need to work through the issues that cause negativity and stress, and train your mind to see only the positive. It is work; I know this and understand the challenge. It takes effort and energy, especially in the beginning, to retrain your thoughts, but it is possible. All things are possible!

Case Study: New Strains of HPV and Your Thoughts

A patient I had worked with previously, and had treated successfully, returned for her annual pap. Her cervix had what appeared to be white pockets of pus on it, but no redness of any sort (for a lot of women, dysplasia appears as red on the cervix). The pap returned as LSIL, which was a new diagnosis for her; she had always been ASGUS if she had an abnormal pap. She had not had any new partners, but my instinct was that she had a new strain of HPV and a very aggressive one at that. I have learned never to ignore my gut feeling when it comes to patient care.

She opted to do the plant treatment again and to only add immune support this time. She added my herbs, and some supplements for the thymus gland that she received from her chiropractor. At the beginning of this cycle of treatment, she was frustrated and a bit afraid that the dysplasia was back, and apparently more aggressive than before; however, I encouraged her to say a positive mantra and to imagine a very healthy cervix. Your cervix looks like a donut (sorry, it does). Pink and beautiful! I tell women that a dysplastic cervix looks like a donut with sprinkles. Imagine the sprinkles going away. One by one, you are picking them off, and pick them off with joy! Imagine a pink donut, maybe with a nice, clear glaze on it. That is what a healthy cervix looks like.

She did all this and, a few months later, we re-papped. The results were completely normal! *Figures 11-15* shows her pap history. She went from having ASGUS with HPV to not having HPV and being normal, to LSIL with HPV again, and then normal. I bring up her case because our body's response to HPV is a very unpredictable.

Clinical Information: 795.01
Repeat pap

DIAGNOSIS
Epithelial Cell Abnormality: Atypical squamous cells of undetermined significance (ASC US)

In this laboratory, a report of atypical squamous cells of undetermined significance indicates approximately a 50% probability of squamous intraepithelial lesion being present on directed biopsy. A number of clinical factors, including high risk HPV status, should be considered in the management of these patients.

Figure 11. ASGUS in 2010.

ACCOUNT:	PATIENT INFORMATION	SPECIMEN INFORMATION
		ACCESSION:
		REQUISITION:
	DOB: AGE:	
	GENDER: F	COLLECTED: 10/04/2010 11:22
PHONE:	ID/MR#:	**RECEIVED: 10/21/2010 06:21**
FAX:	PATIENT PHONE:	REPORTED: 10/25/2010 14:44

CLINICIAN PROVIDED INFORMATION   LAB

HPV DNA, Intermediate/High Risk   Detected   SQL

Infection by high-risk HPV (types 16, 18, 31, 33, 35, 39, 45, 51, 52, 56, 58, 59 or 68) may be associated with precancerous lesions or cancer of the cervix.

Figure 12. HPV in 2010.

	DOB AGE:	
	GENDER: F	COLLECTED: 04/05/2011 NONE
PHONE: 928.214.8793	ID/MR#:	RECIEVED: 04/06/2011 06:46
FAX: 928.214.0147	PATIENT PHONE:	REPORTED: 04/11/2011 11:47

CLINICIAN PROVIDED INFORMATION

DIAGNOSIS
Negative for Intraepithelial Lesion or Malignancy

This is a screening test with an inherent, but low, probability of error. A negative report indicates a high probability of being disease free from squamous cervical cancer and pre-cancer during the next year.

Figure 13. Normal in early 2011.

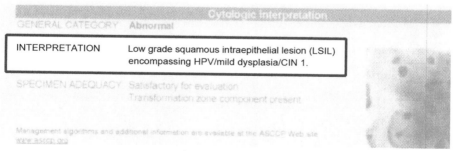

Cytologic interpretation	
GENERAL CATEGORY	Abnormal
INTERPRETATION	Low grade squamous intraepithelial lesion (LSIL) encompassing HPV/mild dysplasia/CIN 1.
SPECIMEN ADEQUACY	Satisfactory for evaluation. Transformation zone component present

Management algorithms and additional information are available at the ASCCP Web site
www.asccp.org

Figure 14. LSIL at the end of 2011.

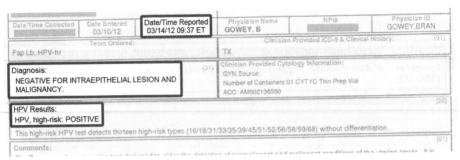

Figure 15. *Normal in early 2012.*

Take Home Messages from this Chapter

1. *I am what I think!*
2. *I should not be afraid to heal toxic emotions. They are not serving me.*

Chapter Nine

Oral Birth Control Use

had successfully treated several patients for cervical dysplsia before I ran into a major roadblock with one who was not improving, even after several months of treatment. Upon further questioning into her history and lifestyle, we reviewed her medication use; she was only taking birth control pills (OCP), which she had been on for years. I had never considered the possibility that birth control pills could cause an abnormal pap smear—but what if this was true?

I suggested she go off them. She was initially hesitant because they decreased menstrual cramps, but I explained that menstrual cramps can be caused by a poor diet, food sensitivities, low magnesium levels, or low Omega 3 levels, all of which we had been working to restore. I felt she most likely would not have a problem with cramps but, if she did, we could do acupuncture or pain medication to help alleviate those. She decided to trust the process and go off the birth control pills.

The results were quick and astounding! Within the next two visits (over a two-month period), her cervix responded quickly to my *Protocol*. It was so fast that I recommended she re-pap with her primary care provider, Sherry Tackett. She did and the results were normal! This occurred 10 weeks after she went off the birth control pills.

This experience prompted me to begin research to see if I could find any link between birth control pill use and abnormal paps. I actually began to find so many articles that I had to stop myself from looking! The highlights of my findings are below, which include a meta-analysis on 52,082 women from 214 studies worldwide that clearly document increased cervical dysplasia with birth control pill use (Fenseca et al. 2011 and Chichareen 2006):

1. **Birth control pills may decrease your body's natural ability to induce cell-death** (called apoptosis) in damaged (cancerous and precancerous) cells. This happens by the OCP's ability to increase expression of specific oncogenes (E6, E7, and HPV16), which then bind to and degrade the genes normally inducing apoptosis, specifically p54 and p53 (Moodley et al. 2003 and Samir et al. 2011).

2. **Birth control pills cause inflammation in cervical cells** by increasing COX-2, the enzyme which suppresses the inflammatory regulator, interleukin-10 (Samir et al. 2011).

3. **Progestin/progesterone-only hormone treatments** cause a 30% higher risk of progression from CIN I to more advanced stages of dysplasia (Gaines et al. 2004 and Hefler et al. 2010).

4. **The longer you use OCPs, the higher your risk** (Gaines et al. 2004).

5. **OCPs cause deficiencies in vitamin B-6.**

I wonder how many primary care physicians and gynecologists are aware of these statistics? I would highly recommend to the medical community that the standard of care changes to screen women for HPV/dysplasia before prescribing OCPs, and fully educating women about the risks involved in using this form of birth control. Generally, at your annual exam, birth control pills are prescribed the day the pap is done, and women are usually not counseled as to risks. Would you choose your method of birth control differently if you knew the results of your pap, or the risks involved with OCPs?

Whether or not to be on birth control pills is still your choice. I do recommend that, if you do all the other things suggested in this book and your pap smears still do not improve, you may want to consider going off the pill or any other form of hormone replacement. Many women on birth control pills fail to use protection with new partners. This increases the risk of contracting HPV. If you are on birth control pills, you should still use protection with new partners. Remember that most men do not have symptoms of HPV and are often carriers of the virus, or they may have other viruses, such as HIV or herpes. Be smart and cautious, and never trust that your new partner does not have HPV, as there is currently no efficacious testing for men.

While I am commenting on contracting HPV from your partner, I want to caution you about contracting what I call a spiritual sexually transmitted disease. When you have intercourse with someone, you are connecting closely energetically, emotionally and, in many respects, spiritually. When a woman opens to her partner, it involves allowing someone else to penetrate her on all these levels (physically, spiritually and emotionally). If you do not like someone's energy, if they are in a place in life that you question, or they are going through emotions and experiences that do not resonate with you, you may want to find a new partner or wait and give yours time to sort things out. As soon as you sleep with someone, you take on that energy. The question is: DO YOU WANT IT?

Case Study: Hormone Replacement/OCP Use

I really wish I had photos of the cervix from this case to show you. Like the patient I mentioned above, this patient also had a dramatic change in her paps after removing hormones from her health regime.

A 54-year-old woman presented to me complaining of cervical dysplasia with HPV. She had been monogamous for years, as she had been married to the same man since she was 30. However, they had recently divorced and she was dating new men. She had not used protection with any of these men, trusting them when they said they were "free of disease".*

*Ladies never trust anyone who says this. I hear from women so often that they decided not to use protection because someone tells them they are "disease-free". It is a mistake that you very much want to avoid making. Remember, MEN USUALLY DO NOT HAVE SYMPTOMS AND THERE IS CURRENTLY NO RELIABLE LAB TESTING FOR THEM! USE A CONDOM WITH NEW PARTNERS!

When this patient was married, she never had abnormal paps, nor did she have HPV. After she was divorced, that changed and new stressors were added to her lifestyle, such as working more and not eating as well. We started her treatment with high-dose oral vitamins, immune support and stress-management techniques (I suggested meditation, art, journaling, and yoga). I encouraged her to find time for herself in her schedule in order to properly focus on her overall health.

After a few months of this protocol, I was not seeing many changes to her cervix. It was not worsening, but it was not getting better, either. We discussed her use of hormone replacement (HRT); she had been on the pill up until the time she started menopause, at which time she went on hormone replacement

Date/Time Collected 04/11/12 00:00 E*	Date Entered 04/12/12	Date/Time Reported 04/17/12 17:00 ET	Physician Name GOWEY, B	NPI#	Physician ID GOWEY,BRAN
	Tests Ordered:		Clinician Provided ICD-9 & Clinical Finding:		
Pap Lb: HPV-hr			622.10 : Dysplasia of cervix, unspecified		
Diagnosis: NEGATIVE FOR NTPAEPITHELIA LESION AND MALIGNANCY.		(p1)	Clinician Provided Cytology Information: GYN Source: Number of Containers: 1 CYTYC Thin Prep Vial ACC: AN292136560		
HPV Results: HPV, high-risk The quality of specimen remaining in the vial after Pap slide preparation was less than the 4 mL minimum cell suspension required. Low sample cellularity may be the cause. See HPV ASR test result. This high-risk HPV test detects thirteen high-risk types (16/18/31/33/35/39/45/51/52/56/58/59/68) without differentiation. HPV, ASR: NEGATIVE					(25.931)

Figure 16. Post-treatment pap results.

therapy. However, she had never had her hormone levels tested prior to going on HRT.

I tested her thyroid and all her adrenal hormones. She had hypothyroidism, so I kept her on her thyroid medication (Levothyroxine), but took her off the hormone replacement. She had some initial symptoms when coming off the hormones, such as hot flashes. In Eastern Medicine terms, hot flashes are due to an energetic deficiency in the chi (energy) of your liver, while from a biochemical, Western perspective, the liver processes hormones before you eliminate them, so there may be a deficiency in a detoxification pathway.

I used a blend of liver herbs for her symptoms. After one month of using the herbs, her hot flashes went away. After two more months of treatment, she had no symptoms related to coming off the hormones. Her cervix began to change for the positive at month three. We watched and waited for three months after that, re-did her pap smear and her results had gone from CIN III to ASGUS.

Three more months later, her pap smear was normal. The final pap results she wanted to share with all of you. See *Figure 16*.

Take Home Messages from this Chapter

1. *I need to consider how long I have been on birth control pills; do I need them?*
2. *I should consider using other forms of birth control, such as condoms.*
3. *I should consider going off all forms of hormones if necessary to heal.*

Chapter Ten

Hormones

To prevent a virus from becoming active on your skin and cause deleterious effects, your internal body has to be strong. I consistently see that women who have low chi (low energy) also have low hormone levels, a phenomenon called "adrenal fatigue".

Your adrenal glands are part of the endocrine system. This is the system that produces and regulates all your hormones, whether that is thyroid hormone, estrogen, testosterone, progesterone, DHEA or pregnenolone. All of the endocrine glands are extremely important; they regulate functions such as your metabolism, weight, water retention, memory and strength. The adrenals are the most overlooked and passed-over glands in the endocrine system, but are the most important (in my opinion). The adrenals are small glands (approximately the size of a walnut) that sit above your kidneys. They take from your body cholesterol and vitamin D and, with that, manufacture most of your hormones (estrogen, DHEA, pregnenalone, testosterone and progesterone, for example). See *Figure 17*.

All the hormones produced by the adrenal glands are important. Estrogen puts on weight, affects the ovulation/menstrual cycle and, in women, has a role in bone health and energy. Testosterone is especially key for men. It regulates their libido, muscle mass, energy level and drive for activities (not just sex). Cortisol is the hormone most people are not as familiar with and will be the focus of this discussion.

Cortisol regulates the following functions:

1. **Blood Sugar/Insulin** (works with insulin to bring sugars into cells)
2. **Sleep/Wake Cycle** (is more powerful to regulate this cycle than melatonin)
3. **Mood** (if too low, cortisol will cause depression and anxiety)
4. **Energy Level** (increases energy levels and stamina)
5. **Aids Absorption of Nutrients** (from the gut)
6. **Memory** (cortisol is needed by the hypothalamus for building memory)
7. **Immune System Regulation** (elevated cortisol suppresses your immune system)
8. **Thyroid Function** (blocks cellular uptake of the thyroid hormone, T3) (Powell 2004)

Normally, cortisol has a daily cycle; it is higher in the morning, then has a few rises and falls during the day before it finally drops at night, allowing you to sleep. The secretion of cortisol by your adrenals is very sensitive to stress, and from any kind of stressor. Under stress, the levels of cortisol initially increase to help you cope with the situation or the thoughts you are having (yes, even thoughts create stress!). The elevated levels send signals to your body to keep your blood sugar levels even while your metabolism slows so as to conserve energy. The problems, however, start when the stress does not stop, or your reaction to the stress does not ease. The cortisol levels will stay high, but they will eventually drop or flip-flop because your body cannot keep up with production of cortisol. I tend to see levels of cortisol that are too low in the morning but may be too high at night, which makes you sluggish (or depressed) when you get up and unable to sleep at night. There is also a tight link between your adrenals and

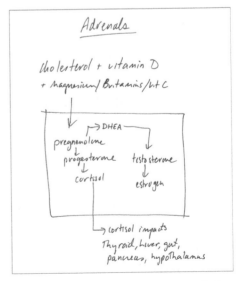

Figure 17. This is a drawing I made for a patients to explain adrenal hormones (Greenspan 1997).

your thyroid. If cortisol elevates it will block your T3, which is the metabolically active form of thyroid hormone. Then a different type of T3 will be made, called "reverse T3" which will slow your metabolism and start to increase your TSH levels (TSH is the main hormone tested when evaluating whether or not you have thyroid disease). If you are struggling with fatigue even though you are on thyroid hormone it may be because you need adrenal support. I have an herbal formulation I created for my patients that helps the adrenals: I love this formula! You can find it on my website.

Testing your adrenal levels is best done with saliva. I use the Diagnos-Techs Adrenal Stress Index (see **Figure 18** for a sample test). I do not use blood tests to measure cortisol; I have not found them to be able to determine adrenal function as effectively as saliva tests. If you feel you need this test, contact your Naturopathic Physician.

Below is an outline of some of the treatments I offer patients for restoring adrenal function. The adrenals require sleep and high levels of vitamins to make hormones. I will describe the benefits of each treatment option below; the key is to pick and choose which is best for you:

1. *Vitamin I.V. Therapies:* These were developed by Dr. Meyer, MD, and now may be called "Meyer's Cocktails", which are high-dose levels of vitamin C mixed with B-vitamins, magnesium, calcium, selenium, zinc and other trace minerals, such as chromium or manganese (see page 11). The standard I.V. bag for a Meyer's Cocktail is rather large at 500 cc and has 30 cc of vitamin C in it. I have found that the large bag is not necessary, as a bag half the size and price works just as well in terms of beneficial outcomes (and doesn't take as long to drip into your veins). A Meyer's Cocktail can take as long as 3 hours; a 250 cc bag can take anywhere from 45 minutes to an hour. I do less vitamin C than a Meyer's, but with the same benefit. High-dose vitamin C can be hard on some patients' veins when infused: another reason for a smaller dose per treatment. That being said, if you have cancer, all the studies point to the benefit of doing a full Meyer's Cocktail with 30 cc of vitamin C. It is important to note that vitamin C is very helpful at detoxifying most molecules, including medications. If you choose to go the route of a full Meyer's Cocktail, make certain your physician is monitoring your symptoms and/or medication levels. I always recommend that you find a Naturopathic Physician in your area, as we tend to specialize in treatments such as these. You can also increase your vitamin levels via diet by eating foods rich in vitamin C (berries), magnesium

Adrenal Stress Index (ASI)

Free Cortisol Values: (nM= Nano Molar)

7:00 AM — 8:00 AM	70	Elevated	13—23
11:00 AM — 12:00 PM	24	Elevated	4—8
4:00 PM — 5:00 PM	12	Elevated	3—8
11:00 PM — 11:59 PM	10	Elevated	1—3

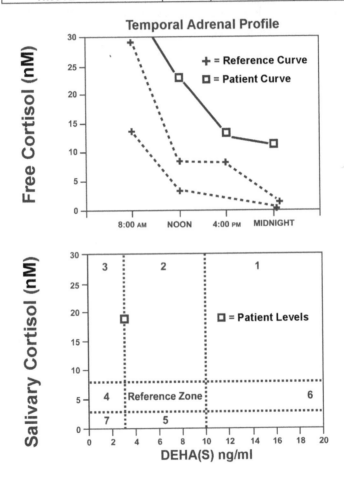

Figure 18. Sample adrenal test, showing the normal rhythm compared to an abnormal cortisol level. This patient is under a lot of stress.

(leafy greens), B-vitamins (meats and nutritional yeast) and trace minerals (greens and veggies).

2. *Adrenal Supportive Supplements*: You have options here, but I am very picky about supplements that really work to support the adrenals. I've only seen a few supplements that affect change in the positive, so, if you take something for the adrenals and you do not feel a difference, do not take that supplement! I used to recommend the Integrative Therapeutics Adrenal Stress End for use in the morning to support the rebuilding of the adrenals, but now I primarily use only my own blend of adrenal herbs (*howdoitreatnaturally.com*) because I have found that herbs rebuild the adrenals in a nourishing, non-stimulating way.

3. *Prescription Adrenal Support*: Hydrocortisone is an option for adrenal support when it is compounded. You will need a prescription from your doctor for this. I only have patients use this option if their adrenal test (via saliva) comes back as completely flat-lined. I also use hydrocortisone for patients who've had their thyroid surgically removed, or have hypothyroidism and are struggling with getting the right thyroid dose. Sometimes, it is that link between adrenals and thyroid that is causing the problem, rather than one gland or the other in isolation.

4. *Sleep*: I know we all hear about this, but it is more important than I can say. Your adrenals require sleep to be restored. I usually recommend to patients that they try to get to bed by 9:00 p.m. and sleep for at least nine hours. Some of us need more sleep than this, and some need less, but, on average, I see that nine hours is optimal. You should be able to wake without an alarm and, when you get enough sleep with a regular bedtime, this is possible. It is also wise to incorporate exercise, time for yourself, time for reflection, or time for the arts, to help reduce and manage your stress.

I know most of my colleagues will test estrogen, progesterone and testosterone levels, and, if the levels come back as low, they will put patients on hormone replacement. Most colleagues will have a compounding pharmacy put all these hormones together. I have noticed that some women metabolize progesterone to cortisol when progesterone is used topically, so I do not recommend it to be used this way; progesterone is best taken orally. I have also learned that general adrenal support—since all these hormones are made in the adrenal gland—does oftentimes restore the levels of the other hormones (estrogen, progesterone or testosterone). In other words, you may not need HRT (hormone replacement therapy) if you treat the adrenal glands with adrenal herbs and nutrition.

Case Study: Balancing Adrenal/Thyroid

This is a case that is not related to HPV, but it very powerfully illustrates the importance of treating your hormonal system with respect.

A patient presented with extreme fatigue, weight loss, dark circles under her eyes, memory loss, depression, a lack of will and weakness. She had recently been diagnosed with thyroid cancer, among other conditions, and had her thyroid removed.

Post surgery, she had been put on Synthroid (a type of thyroid medication). It seemed to work for a while, but then she started to go through a lot of stress in her life—from financial worries to relationship and job issues. She was struggling with staying focused and on-task at work, she felt lackluster, and was very weak and underweight.

At first, it seemed like we only needed a different thyroid medication. I usually use Nature-throid, which is a balance of T4, T3 and has some T2. Some patients do better on Nature-throid as opposed to Synthroid (another thyroid medication that is just T4) or other medications, so we switched her medication. She felt great at first, but then started to take a dive in how she felt. Again, I checked her labs and switched the dose ever so slightly. By this time, she was so thin and weak that I also added the vitamin I.V. drips to her treatment. Her skin was becoming increasingly dry (typical for people with thyroid problems), and she was very dehydrated even though she was drinking water (also typical problem for people with thyroid problems). With every I.V. treatment we did, and with every slight change in her thyroid dose, she improved only slightly, but then crashed again.

After a few months of this, it finally dawned on me that I needed to balance her thyroid with her adrenals. There is such a close association between these glands that it is difficult to treat one without the other.

I had a compounding pharmacist make a blended adrenal glandular (hydrocortisone, a little estrogen, testosterone and progesterone) with the thyroid medication. You would not believe how this woman turned around. She went from being so thin it scared me to being beautiful, strong and healthy. She had been on disability but, after a few months of this treatment, she went back to work! After a bit more time, she was off the estrogen/testosterone/progesterone and just using my adrenal herbs as a supplement with her thyroid medication.

Take Home Messages from this Chapter

1. *I need to balance my hormonal system! Herbals are one way to do that, but I have many options.*
2. *Naturopathic Doctors are experts in balancing hormones and specialize in treating the adrenals.*
3. *I probably need more sleep than I think I need.*

Chapter Eleven

Smoking's Not All
It's Cracked Up to Be

I t is well documented that smoking is very hard on cervical cells. In 1977, Winkelstein Jr., was the first to put smoking as a risk factor to a testable hypothesis. He found it is a risk factor even when other variables are removed and studies from 2003-2010 have all confirmed this. While no expert agrees fully as to why, the general idea is that the DNA of cervical cells changes with exposure to nicotine or the by-products of nicotine; or, free radical damage caused by the nicotine/chemicals within cigarette smoke causes changes on a cellular level. Cervical mucus has several measurable amounts of cigarette constituents and metabolites within including benzo(a), nicotine and pyrene.

Here are some findings in the literature:

- *Pyrenes may increase intake of HPV into cervical cells.*
- *Nicotine inhibits apoptosis (cell death of damaged cells), causes cellular proliferation, or stimulates endothelial growth factor.*
- *Smokers have less T cells, NK (natural killer cells), helper T cells and lower levels of IgGs.*
- *Exposure to smoke causes changes in DNA expression (in genes DNMT1, DNMT3A, DNMT3B).*

- *Smoke suppresses tumor suppression gene, P16, which is highly associated in women with CIN II and CIN III.*
- *Smoking causes "polymorphisms", which are changes to genes when exposed to a chemical.*
- *Smoking cigarettes and marijuana increases immune suppression versus cigarette smoking alone (Fenesca et al. 2011).*

I have not personally worked with any patients who've had cervical dysplsia and were smokers, so I do not have any clinical stories to share at this time. However, the studies that do exist on the correlation between cigarette smoking, cervical dysplasia and cancer are very clear. I do recommend that anyone who is struggling with a history of abnormal paps and is a smoker to consider quitting, or those who are regularly exposed to cigarette smoke find ways of avoiding it. If you cannot quit, I would then recommend that you see your gynecologist for any of the procedure options that treat abnormal paps, including the LEEP. If you do quit smoking, or lessen your second-hand exposure to cigarette smoke, I recommend that you read the chapter (see *Chapter 2*) on environmental toxins and purchase one of the FIR Infrared Saunas, use it regularly, and add high doses of antioxidants to your daily intake.

Take Home Messages from this Chapter

1. *Cigarette by-products can be found in cervical cells.*
2. *Smoking is linked to abnormal pap results.*
3. *Cigarette smoke causes DNA changes.*

Chapter Twelve

Viral Diseases in General

treat a lot of viral diseases, such as hepatitis (hep A, hep B, hep C), CMV, Epstein-Barr and influenza. Viruses often cause the following symptoms:

Fatigue (often very extreme)
Joint pain/swelling
Rashes (they often come and go, but usually show up before other symptoms)
Low-grade fever
Diarrhea
Pain
Swelling of major organs (i.e., liver or spleen)
Memory loss
Body aches
Depression/anger
Swollen lymph nodes
Changes to appetite
Irregular heartbeat

Physicians often miss the diagnosis of a viral infection because the symptoms can and do look like so many other diseases. Viral diseases can be tricky to treat (as you are learning by reading this book), but it is not impossible. You may always have the virus, but you do not always have to have problems. Below is an excerpt from a phone message a patient left on February 23, 2012, after she had worked with me on treating abnormal paps and herpes:

> I want you to know I am 12 weeks pregnant. My blood work and everything is perfect and I wanted to call you and thank you because I probably would not have gotten this far without your help. So, thank you. — L., New Jersey

In general, you need to treat any virus just as you would HPV:

1. Avoid processed sugars.
2. Do castor oil packs over your liver.
3. Eat lots of vegetables and good sources of protein.
4. Stay alkaline.
5. Do alternating hot/cold treatments to affected joints and/or your abdomen to increase immune cell levels and activity.

Diet is especially key for patients with hepatitis induced by viruses. **DO NOT EAT SUGAR!** See the next case study if you don't believe me.

Case Study: Hepatitis C

A patient presented to me with long-standing pain and swelling in his hands and feet. He had been to "all the doctors", and none had any answers for him. In fact, his treatment protocol from his physician was to "come back in twelve years", which, to his sister and mother, meant he would die from the hepatitis.

After taking his entire history, I studied his medical records. My first instinct was that he had a viral infection, as swelling of extremities accompanied by pain may be caused by a virus, especially if it is preceded by a rash or illness (which it had been, although that had occurred months beforehand). When looking through his records, I noticed that a previous physician had run blood work for hepatitis C and he was positive for it. That being said, no one had told him he had hepatitis.

The family took him back to see the doctor they had been working with, who told them that hepatitis would in no way cause joint pain or swelling. I was very surprised to hear this. Regardless, I began immune supportive and nutritional treatments with him. Below is a summary of what I prescribed:

1. Xymogen IgG
2. Mother Nature's Immune Blend (my formula)
3. Vitamin I.V. drips
4. Alternating hot/cold treatments to abdomen
5. Castor oil packs over the liver and to hands
6. Acupuncture
7. No processed sugars in diet
8. Mountain Peaks Chronic Immune and Liv C Formulations
9. Homeopathy, as needed

His viral load went from over 6 million to around 3 million in three months with the above treatment. He began to feel better almost immediately; his family felt it was the vitamin I.V.s that worked the best.

We backed off on some of the supplements at about month-6 and retested his viral load. It had gone up again even though he was feeling great and the swelling in his hands and feet were going down. I asked what was different and they admitted they had gotten excited because he was doing so well that they had stopped the castor oil packs, the alternating hot/cold treatments, and he had been eating some sugar again. This was a huge learning experience for all of us, but especially for me. When you are in medical school, you learn that herbs and some supplements have "anti-viral" properties, and, in your mind, you think it means the viral load is dropping like flies or that the virus is getting killed off because of the herbs and supplements. What if viruses stay with us but may not be a problem if we take really good care of ourselves? I told the family to get him off sugar. I retested him almost two months later and his viral load had dropped dramatically (see *Figures 19* and *20*).

Case Study: Chicken Pox

I had a patient call me recently, wondering if her daughter may have contracted the chicken pox from her grandfather, who recently had an acute shingles outbreak (shingles

Figure 19. *Patient on sugars.*

Figure 20. *Patient off sugar, viral load 2 million lower.*

is caused by the same virus as chicken pox). I examined the child and concluded that, yes, she did indeed have chicken pox. The child was about six-months-old and very healthy, as her mother followed all of my preventative medical advice. We did a good multi-vitamin (liquid), essential oils, probiotics and kept her away from foods her mom is sensitive to, so as to avoid any unwanted reactions. We increased the probiotics and added a bit of my immune tincture, properly diluted, with some tips on keeping the lesions dry.

The mother called me later that day and said that, within four hours of dosing her child with the herbs, the lesions were beginning to crust over. Four hours. Think about that for a moment. This is a very healthy child because of the very, very simple things I prescribed to build a healthy immune system (vitamins, probiotics), cell membranes (the fish oils), and gut lining (probiotics and avoiding foods she may be sensitive to). Then, when the right blend of herbs are added, the child's immune system responded quickly.

The mother was so impressed that her child was improving so quickly, she took her to daycare with her sister, who was almost two-years-old. She told the school her younger daughter was recovering from the chicken pox, successfully, and the school administration reacted like she had a life-threatening illness. It was such a strong reaction that the school isolated the older daughter, even though she did not have any signs of the pox. They actually put her in a corner. When the mother went to pick up her daughter she was sitting alone and was very sad.

Why does our society react in such a way? I feel we need to be reacting to our lifestyle as the life-threatening illness: we eat too much sugar, do not exercise adequately, and we eat foods that are bad for us, even though we know we should avoid them. The problem is the way we treat out bodies!

Take Home Messages from this Chapter

1. *Viruses are not impossible to heal from, but they do take a bit of effort and commitment on behalf of the patient.*
2. *Viral load will increase with processed sugar in the diet.*
3. *Viruses can cause symptoms easy to miss by my physician.*

Chapter Thirteen

Gowey Protocol® Gel

I use a proprietary blend of extracts of carnivorous plants *(Sarracenia purpurea* and *flava)* for the **Gowey Protocol® Gel** treatment. Studies done by the University of Wisconsin found that carnivorous plants shrink tumors (Miles and Kokpol 1976). These plants also have measurable amounts of compounds called anthocyanins that are known to induce apoptosis (cell death) in damaged cells (Sheridan 2001).

Many women have a cervix that is easily observable and identifiable via a vaginal speculum exam (the speculum is the tool used in the pap exam to open the vagina). However, a good number of women have a cervix that is curved under, pressed to the side or downward, making it difficult to reach. I am looking for someone to design a medical device for application of the **Gel** onto the cervix; if you know of anyone who could help please have them contact me.

The plant cannot be relied on exclusively; you do need to follow all the other advice I have outlined in this book. If you want your doctor to do this **Protocol**, please have them contact me. I work one-on-one with physicians to teach them the **Protocol**. I also know that Medicine is an Art. Your physician may want to do applications to the cervix other than the **Gowey Protocol® Gel**. *That being said, you are responsible for your healing. I recommend you take seriously the information I have provided in this book to finding your Obstacle to Cure, and start your work there.*

Do not expect results overnight. I have learned from experience that the cervix heals slowly. You have to remember these cells are very delicate, as they are designed to divide rapidly when it is time to deliver a child. Women who are positive about their life, their future, and have an excited outlook on life and on healing, are the ones who heal the fastest.

See Appendixes A and B for my initial case studies and clinical trial using the *Gowey Protocol® Gel*.

Chapter Fourteen

Gowey Protocol® and You

With each patient, I do a full health history during their initial exam. We discuss all the aspects of the patient's health (diet, nutrition, stress, mind/body, environmental toxins, etc.), and then we look together to see areas in the patient's life that may be deficient.

During this process, the patient and I begin to learn where the deficiency (the Obstacle to Cure) is. I can see the changes (or no changes) on the cervix that match what we are learning. For example, if someone is low in their immune system and we add the right immune support, I will see positive changes (i.e., less redness on the cervix). If not, the cervix will not change. The patient will start to look healthier, have greater energy, and will start to understand and know what makes them feel better and what does not. The emotional needs of the patient start to surface more than before, allowing us to start to handle things that have been challenges.

The emotional aspect is really the most important. As women, we energetically want to reach into the community of our lives to fix everyone and everything, while, at the same time, ignoring (not purposefully) our own needs. Or, we try to impose our needs on someone else, making them responsible for our happiness.

It is important to deal with the things that have made you feel unhappy and alone, or stressed. Find your community, and work to bring happiness to others. Your happiness will be met if you trust life enough to let go, and not try to control outcomes.

Take Home Messages from this Chapter

1. *We all have a "weak spot" in our health. This "weakness" may be my obstacle to cure.*
2. *Emotional health is key.*
3. *The cervix can heal. My cervix will heal!*

Chapter Fifteen

The Gowey Protocol® Gel and Squamous Cell Carcinoma

I had a patient who came to me for a recent injury to the bridge of her nose; she had fallen and hit her nose while she was wearing her glasses. The glasses had caused an abrasion on her skin that was concerning to her, so she came to ask me to take a look at it. I made some general recommendations on wound care, instructing her to follow-up with me in two weeks if it did not improve.

She returned promptly after two weeks and the lesion was still there. She wondered if I had anything she could put topically on her skin to induce healing. For some reason, my **Gel** came to mind, so I prescribed some to her with the instructions to schedule a biopsy with a dermatologist. We thought that something might have gotten lodged into her skin during the impact of her fall.

The dermatologist did indeed find small shards of metal in her skin, removed them, and did a biopsy. The biopsy results showed squamous cell carcinoma! She had not yet started to use my **Gel**, as she was waiting for the results of the biopsy.

I told her to schedule the Moh's (which is the standard procedure for removing squamous cell carcinoma from the skin), and, in the meantime, to try the **Gel** as the earliest she could get in for the Moh's was three weeks later. Time is always of the essence when treating cancer, if only for the patient's emotional well-being.

At the three-week visit, the dermatologist was not able to find any sign of the cancer. He re-biopsied the area and the results came back normal. He could not believe the results and cancelled the Moh's procedure.

I have many more cases of patients who were scheduled for an excision of a squamous cell lesion but, in the meantime, wanted me to prescribe some of the **Gowey Protocol® Gel**. By the time they had their follow-up appointment with their dermatologist, there was no lesion on their skin. In fact, in many cases the lesion had gotten crusty and had fallen off; and in some patients, the dermatologist did not re-biopsy because they could not find a lesion to biopsy.

Take Home Messages from this Chapter

1. *As a physician, it is my duty to inform you that the standard of care of squamous cell carcinoma is removal of the lesion via excision (biopsy); the reason is that this type of cancer tends to spread. I am not telling you to avoid this procedure, nor am I telling you to avoid your dermatologist. I am not telling you anything other than case reports of how the Gel has helped more than cervical dysplasia. It is your decision as to where you go from here with this information, but do not neglect discussing anything you decide to pursue in terms of treatment with your physician.*

2. *I should discuss everything with my physician.*

Chapter Sixteen

The Gowey Protocol®
Gel and Warts

've had a few patients who complained of plantar warts and warts on their hands that did not go away, or would come and go. HPV is usually related as the cause of these warts. Common treatment for warts is excision (removal), burning or freezing them off. Alternative medical practitioners will recommend things such as covering the lesions in duct tape, taking the homeopathic thuja or specific dietary changes.

One patient in particular, who had a few warts on the heel of her right foot, was very excited to try the **Gel**. I instructed her to apply the **Gel**, then keep the area covered with a bandage. She did just that, and we followed up every few weeks. The warts actually started to dry up, then they crusted over and, finally, they fell off completely, root and all. Within two months, they were gone.

Another patient was not as lucky. He had a wart on a surface of his penis, which had started a few days after intercourse with a new partner. We tested the lesion via a skin scraping and it was HPV-positive. He has been applying the **Gel** to it for a year and it is slowly improving. He had tried anti-viral medications and topical prescription medications for the wart prior to working with me, but none of those treatments worked for him. He ended up having the wart burned off. I have been reading various articles coming out on Medscape (a physician resource) connecting HPV with penile cancers in men. This virus does not limit its effects to women.

Take Home Messages from this Chapter

1. *Dr. Gowey's Protocol may treat warts.*
2. *Men are affected by HPV and should follow the lifestyle advise in this book to help them heal HPV-related lesions.*

Chapter Seventeen

The Gowey Protocol®
Gel and MRSA

The mother of a five-year-old called me on November 23, 2010, asking for treatment for the antibiotic-resistant skin infection called "MRSA" for her son. He'd had a lesion the size of a quarter on his right thumb for five days. He was put on antibiotics, but the mother was worried because he'd had this before and it took a very long time for him to heal; the antibiotics were very hard on the boy's gut, tending to cause multiple adverse reactions.

I had seen the **Gowey Protocol® Gel** help other skin lesions, so I asked her if she wanted to try it. She agreed and I prescribed it for her son. I tried to reach her a few times via phone after this initial visit, and was finally able to reach her on December 14, 2010. She shared that her son's skin started to heal within 24 hours of the application of the **Gel**. She said, "As soon as I put the **Gel** formula on his skin, it started to heal and I took him off antibiotics the next day!"

At the time of writing this book, I am working towards starting clinical trials to evaluate the efficacy of the **Gowey Protocol® Gel** on MRSA skin lesions. Please refer back to my website (*howdoitreatnaturally.com*) for the posting of the results of that study, or sign up for my newsletter; I will send out alerts as new information is posted.

Take Home Messages from this Chapter

1. *Dr. Gowey's Gel works on many different skin lesions, not just cervical dysplasia.*
2. *MRSA is a type of skin infection that antibiotics do not generally treat.*
3. *Just because I may have a condition conventional medicine cannot treat does not mean there are not options available.*

Conclusion

Identify Your
Obstacle to Cure

Everyone has a weak spot in their health; whether it's your immune system, an inability to absorb nutrients well, a negative living situation, exposure to environmental toxins, or a combination of all of the above, we each have something that is an obstacle to cure. Naturopathic Medicine is not about treating symptoms with "natural remedies"; it is about identifying and treating causes (the obstacle to cure), and then using the right medications, diet or supplements to support healing.

You need to work with your physician to find the cause of your illness or dis-ease, then, treat the cause. Every disease has this common root. Find it and be well. For every person, there is a perfectly fitted physician—someone who knows your health history and will always look deeper. Naturopathic Physicians are trained to look deeper, and that is something that I love most about what we do.

Use this time on your journey through the *Protocol* to develop deep self-love. One thing I have learned over time is the importance of self-love, of looking inward for everything that you need, for not projecting your needs onto others, for standing strong within yourself and for looking inward to find your special gifts to bring out into the world. My lessons in this catapulted when I lost my dearest brother to a motorcycle accident in June of 2010. We were very close.

Losing him left me feeling very empty inside, sometimes angry, sometimes frustrated, and in a state of not understanding how the Universe works. But, through it all, I feel I have been given the gift of knowing myself better, and I encourage you to use the setbacks in your life to do the same. Part of my *Protocol* is learning to love you, and be okay with yourself no matter what happens in your life.

Dr. Brandie Gowey was able to help me by diagnosing my health problems and completely correcting my entire system—when no other doctor or meds could. She is an amazing doctor who truly listens and cares about her patients; she shows you how to achieve and maintain the best possible health by balancing your system and your body to help you feel well from the inside out, helping you find the best possible version of yourself.
— A., Flagstaff, AZ

Be well, ladies, be well. You deserve the best, most abundant and healthy life. Fight for it, as it is well worth it. And please know that I am always here for you. Your cervix can heal. I have patients that are living proof of that. If you have cancer from HPV or are a cancer survivor, I am not making light or less of your situation. I understand. What I am saying is that we have more power over our health than we realize, much of it is a choice. And, it is about educating yourself so that you can start to find your obstacle to any kind of "cure". Take your time with your healing; it is definitely a process as learning about yourself takes time.

I believe in you!

Initial Consultation Checklist

This checklist will help you determine your **OBSTACLE TO CURE** within the **Gowey Protocol®**. Use it during your initial consultation with your physician.

Please circle **yes** or **no** responses questions where appropriate or *fill-in-the blanks*.

1a. Do you live in a large city (yes or no)?
1b. Do you spend time outdoors in this city (yes or no)?
*1c. Where were you born?*_____

If you were born in a polluted area, or an area known for certain pollutants, you may have higher than normal levels of toxins stored within in your cells. Everyone has toxins, but not everyone has a problem with them. Some people detoxify easily and some do not. See *Chapter 2*.

Suggestions:

• Get an infrared sauna (FIR) and do 20-30 minutes a few days a week, followed by a cold rinse. This is the best type of sauna to use to detoxify.
• Do castor oil packs over your liver.
• Body brush.
• Eat high levels of anti-oxidant rich foods.
• Try to avoid chemical use/solvent exposure as from salon products/paint/exhaust fumes.

2a. Do you eat sugary foods (yes or no)?
2b. Do you eat sugary foods regularly (yes or no)?

Please do not eat any sugary foods, and if you do, eat very little. Sugar suppresses your immune system and depletes your body of important nutrients such as magnesium. See *Chapters 5* and *12*.

3. What do you eat most regularly? List these foods in the space below:

_____

_____

_____

_____

If you are seeing more protein or processed foods than veggies you are most likely too acidic (in body tissues). You can get pH paper and test your urine to see what your pH is exactly. Ideally it is around 6.5. If it is below 5, you are too acidic and you need to eat more alkalinizing foods. Eating more veggies and bright colored fruits also increases your total body load of antioxidants, which are necessary for signaling to diseased cells to die off, a process called "apoptosis". See *Chapters 2, 5, 6* and *7*.

4. Food sensitivities

Everyone has foods they are sensitive to; by eating them, an inflammatory reaction is triggered. If the inflammation persists, your cervical cells will be unable to clear the effects of the HPV. You can do a food sensitivity panel: I use Immunolabs as they test all 4 subtypes of inflammatory cells that respond to foods; or, you can do an elimination diet (take out one food at a time, the most common foods you eat) and wait 2 weeks to see any changes in how you feel; it takes at least 9 days for inflammatory reactions to calm. Your physician will know you are taking out the right foods by positive changes on your cervix. See *Chapter 5*.

I took _____ out of my diet and *I Feel Better!* (Wheat, dairy, soy, sugar, eggs, and cranberries are some of the most common foods that cause inflammation.)

5a. Do you get colds/flu easily/often (yes or no)?

5b. Do you have any other viral related diseases such as HIV or herpes (yes or no)?

If you tend to get sick often or have other viral diseases that are chronic you need to support your immune system. The herbs I formulated for this purpose are excellent, some of the best quality herbs around (see my website for the Immune Blend—Mother Nature's Remedy). They are liquid, the taste is strong for some people but you can dilute them before you take some.

There are various pathways by which your immune system can and does regulate your response to viral cells. Special types of T cells called "helpers", or Th1, do this. They, however, can become overshadowed by the effects of toxins in our environment, pushing another type of T helper cell, called Th2. You may want to integrate the detoxifying suggestions I make, to help promote more Th1. The herbs will also help you do this.

If you do all this and do not improve, please have your physician do the **Genova test**. It is a genetic test that looks at which immune pathways your body pro-motes. The test, around $250, is well worth the investment. The information will aid in making a specific treatment for you. See *Chapters 7* and *12*.

6a. Do you drink alcohol regularly (yes or no)?
6b. Do you smoke cigarettes (yes or no)?
6c. Do you have a lot of stress in your life (yes or no)?
6d. Do you feel supported in your life by family/friends (yes or no)?
If you answered yes to any of these questions you need to:

- *Stop smoking*
- *Drink alcohol less often*
- *Incorporate stress management into your lifestyle*
- *Find a support network, even something as simple as joining a YMCA and getting active in their classes may make you feel more connected to community.*

Stress, alcohol, and smoking all deplete your body of key nutrients. You need these nutrients to kick the HPV; smoking by-products are stored in your cervical cells, making you more susceptible to developing abnormal changes on your cervix. See *Chapters 8* and *11*.

7a. Do you use birth control (yes or no)?

7b. Do you use hormone replacement (yes or no)?

7c. Do you have intercourse with new partners without condoms?

There is no test currently for men for HPV. You need to use condoms, especially with new partners or you run the risk of acquiring new strains of the virus.

Hormones activate genes within cervical cells that make you more susceptible to HPV. Discuss other forms of birth control with your physician and consider using adrenal herbs instead of HRT creams/individual hormones. My adrenal herbs were created for this purpose and support the gland that makes all those hormones (the adrenal glands) as a whole. See *Chapters 4, 9* and *10.*

8a. Do you have a family history of cervical cancer (yes or no)?

You may be more susceptible to HPV so you may need to do all the above. See *Chapter 6.*

9. Do you find yourself thinking or saying negative things?

Your body hears every word you say! You need to say all day long, *"I am healthy, I am whole, I am beautiful and my cervix is perfect!"* Write down positive statements on pieces of paper and put them where you will always see them (on your bathroom mirror or in your car, for example). Keep saying it (out loud and to yourself) and your body and spirit will eventually believe it! See *Chapter 8.*

I have all patients use 6-8 grams of the plant **Gel** nightly unless they are menstruating. I use _____ grams a night, or my Physician has me using _____vaginal application _____ nightly.

Appendix A

Limiting the Deleterious Effects of the Herpes Simplex Virus, a Phase II Clinical Trial
Dr. Brandie Gowey, NMD
Gowey Research Group, PLLC

Abstract: *Sarracenia purpurea* (pitcher plant) is an anti-viral herb used historically as a "cure" (*webmd.com*) for small pox (Chalmers 1862). HSV I and II is a viral disease affecting millions of patients globally with vesicular lesions that can be very painful and can last for weeks to months before they resolve, tending to manifest on mucosal membranes. Preliminary case reports by the author revealed that topical use of *S. purpurea*, when compounded in an aloe-based **Gel** manufactured by Professional Compounding Centers of America, gave patients immediate relief from pain caused by the virus; and within two to seven days, lesions were resolved or resolving fully. In this double-blind, placebo-controlled study, patients with recent (within 48 hours) outbreaks of HSV I and II lesions were given the compounded *S. purpurea* extract or placebo, and applied either formulation directly to the lesions every three to four hours. Lesion number, size, and severity of pain were measured. Outcomes were statistically significant at $p < 0.05$, demonstrating possible effectiveness within two days of *S. purpurea* against HSV I and II.

Background: Herpes Simplex (HSV) is a viral infection with two subtypes, I and II, that cause painful, vesicular lesions on skin or mucosal membranes, affecting 50 million in the United States alone (*uptodate.com*). Herpes lesions tend to manifest on oral or genital membranes, although they have been found to erupt on almost any external tissue. The virus remains dormant on the dorsal root ganglion, travels up the peripheral nerves to the local tissue, and causes vesicles that can last six weeks or longer. Herpes outbreaks are precipitated by stress, co-infection, trauma, sun exposure, fever, or low nutritional levels. HSV antibodies are detectable in 30% of patients in high socioeconomic groups and in nearly 100% of low, while a large majority of cases are not clinically apparent (meaning antibodies are not detectable). Diagnosis is generally made via clinical history and physical examination, although lab tests, such as viral culture, remains the gold-standard to identify the virus; serum titers may identify the presence of IgGs or IgMs. Conventional treatment of the virus includes oral antiviral medications, such as Acyclovir, with long-term dosing of one year or longer. Current Naturopathic treatment includes immune system support, topical lysine (an amino acid that inhibits viral growth), vitamin therapy, or antiviral herbs. Current OTC treatments can take two weeks or longer to relieve symptoms, and most of these treatments have not been verified with clinical trials (*mdconsult.com*). *Sarracenia purpurea* is a carnivorous plant native to the wetlands of most of the eastern United States and Canada; its vast range makes it the most common and broadly distributed pitcher plant, even though most of its habitat has been destroyed. The plant's leaves are modified into cups that look like pitchers, and it is these "pitchers" that secrete a sweet nectar, attracting insects (Rice 2005). Insects get trapped in the bottom of the pitcher and then are digested by bacteria in the juice. Compounds in these pitchers are anthocyanins, such as delphinidin or cyanidin. Anthocyanincs are known in nature for their anti-oxidant, anti-viral and apoptosis properties (*wikipedia. org/wiki/anthocyanins*).

An extensive literature review was conducted to assess medicinal value of *S. purpurea*. Limited information was found, with most references on related species (Miles and Kokpol 1974 and 1976), or on its effects against small pox (Chalmers 1862). Most references call the pitcher plant a stimulating tonic, diuretic and laxative. The root is thought to be helpful in relieving some gastric problems, or any "torpid condition of the stomach, the intestines, the liver, the kidneys, or the uterus" (*Henriette's Herbal* 2010), possibly also reducing scar formation (*webmd.com*). Thus far, only one modern drug (Sarapin) has been FDA approved from the pitcher plant and manufactured for the treatment of neuromuscular or neuralgic pain (Rice 2005). It appears, however, that without new research, the plant will generally continue to be thought of as "completely obsolete" (LaGow 2004).

Purpose of Study: The purpose of this study was to substantiate the clinical ability of a compounded *S. purpurea* (**Gowey Protocol® Gel**) extract to resolve lesions caused by HSV I and II, within two days. Markers such as pain, size of lesions and duration of symptoms were evaluated relative to placebo; patients were followed over the course of two weeks, and presented to clinic on Days 1, 3, 5 and 14. Methods and Design: Men and women ages 18 and up experiencing a current herpes outbreak (within three days of onset of symptoms) were recruited via newspaper ads per IRB consent. Thirty-three patients enrolled in the study, which was conducted from January 2011 to March 2011, with nine degrees of freedom. Patients who had a previous diagnosis confirmed by their primary care doctor were enrolled. Patients excluded from the study were those who were pregnant, had risk of herpetic encephalitis, widespread infection of herpes, were currently using antiviral medications or who did not have a current outbreak. Patients were seen at the Naturopaths International (*nimobile.org*) clinic in Flagstaff, Arizona. Patients were screened on Day 1 for active lesions and exclusion criteria. If they qualified to participate, they were instructed as to any possible side effects and/or risks of enrolling in the study, and informed consent was obtained as well as release of information for use in furthering research. Permission to obtain photos was also obtained. Patients were assigned randomly placebo or active, unknown to patient and researcher. **Gel** was applied to lesions every three to four hours in a small amount to cover the lesion, and patients returned on Days 3, 5, and 14. Photos of lesions were taken on patients who gave permission; size of lesions were measured as well as number and subjective pain scale 1-10, with 10 being the worse pain possible. This data was recorded and tracked for statistical purposes. ANOVA, two-tailed tests were used to evaluate patient data.

Intervention: Patients were given a ¼ oz tube of either active **Gel** or placebo. They applied the **Gel** every three to four hours in an amount enough to cover the lesions over the course of two weeks.

Outcome measures: For the 33 patients enrolled in this clinical trial, the mean and standard deviation values for diameter of lesion (in mm) and pain scale were calculated for Days 1, 3, 5 and 14. Mean values were similar on the first day for both active (**Gel**) and placebo, at 8.2/8.3 and 6.1/4.1 respectively. However, by Day 3, there was nearly a 50% drop in lesion diameter for active group (to 4.2), while the placebo actually increased slightly (to 8.4). The active group continued to see a drop in lesion diameter to 1.5 mm and 0.2 mm by Days 5 and 14. Pain rating showed a significant drop, from 6.1 to 0.2 in the active group by Day 3, and to 0.0 for the duration of the study. In contrast, placebo group showed an increase in pain by day 3 (from 4.1 to 4.7), dropped slightly to 4.6 by day 5 and to 1.7 by the conclusion of the study (Day 14). See below. Standard deviations from the mean (with n-22 for active group and n-11 for placebo) are also calculated below, and were used to obtain the t value.

Visits	Day 1	Day 3	Day 5	Day 14
Mean Lesion Diameter by Visit				
Active	8.2	4.2	1.5	0.2
Placebo	8.3	8.4	6.9	5.4
Mean Pain Scale by Visit				
Active	6.1	0.2	0.0	0
Placebo	4.1	4.7	4.6	1.7
Standard Deviation Lesion Diameter by Visit				
Active	6.4	4.1	2.2	1.2
Placebo	2.9	3.0	3.4	3.1
Standard Deviation Pain Scale by Visit				
Active	2.7	0.7	0.2	0
Placebo	2.0	3.5	3.4	1.8

Number of lesions were totaled for both active and placebo groups and can be summarized as follows: Patients with the active had the same number of lesions at Days 1 and 3 (25 total), but by Day 5 numbers dropped 60% (to 10) while the placebo group saw an increase in the number of lesions from Days 1 to 3 (from 13 to 15) and again from Day 5 to 14 (from 14 to 15 total).

Results

A two-tailed test was used to evaluate results, with patient outcomes compared on standard bar graphs. This clinical trial was performed to evaluate the effectiveness in a compounded pitcher plant extract formulation (*Gowey Protocol® Gel*) on HSV I and II lesions within two days versus placebo. The data shows that, for lesion diameter and pain, there is a significant reduction in symptoms ($p < .05$), while there was no change in number (frequency) of lesions for the active group (within two days).

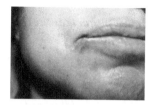

Day 1 of study. *New outbreak of HSV I or II (or both).*

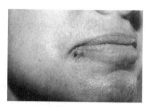

Day 3 of study. *Lesion beginning to crust over.*

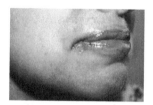

Day 5 of study. *Lesion healing.*

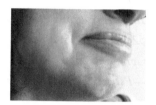

Day 14 of study. *Lesion gone.*

Therefore, the results are significant for lesion diameter and pain and unlikely due to chance. See photos on pages 88 and 89 for images from a patient who gave permission for her photos to be utilized for the purpose of this study.

Conclusions

The **Gowey Protocol® Gel** is an effective treatment for lesions caused by HSV I and II, reducing symptoms within two days of application verses placebo. Considering the limited treatments available for HSV I and II, and the significant social stigma and embarrassment caused by breakouts, the **Gowey Protocol® Gel** mixture deserves further study, so as to evaluate constancy of results as well as to refute arguments made in published literature the lack of merit of the pitcher plant, despite its previous use in treatment of small pox.

References

Chalmers, Miles. *The Employment of Sarracenia Purpurea, or Indian Pitcher Plant, as a Remedy for Small Pox.* **The Lancet.** 1862. p 430-431.

LaGow, Bette. **PDR for Herbal Medicines.** Thompson; Montvale, NJ. 2004.

mdconsult.com

Miles DH and Kokpol U. *Tumor inhibitors II: constituents and antitumor activity of Sarracenia flava.* **J Pharm Sci**. 1976. Feb; 65(2): 284-5.

Miles DH, Kokpol U, et al. T*umor inhibitors. I. Preliminary investigation of antitumor activity of Sarracenia flava.* **J Pharm Sci**. 1974. Apr; 63(4): 613-5.

Pitcher Plant—Sarracenia Purpurea. At: *bio.brandeis.edu/fieldbio/medicinal_plants/pages/Pitcher_Plant.htm.* 2009.

Rice, Barry. *The Carnivorous Plant FAQ—Medicinal.* At: *sarracenia.com/faq/faq1680.html.* 2005.

Rice, Barry. *The Carnivorous Plant FAQ—Sarracenia Overview.* At: *sarracenia.com/faq/faq5520.html.* 2005.

Sarapin. Sarapin.com. 2005.

Sarracenia.—Pitcher Plant. At: *henrieteesherbal.com/eclectic/kings/sarracenia.html.* 2009.

Slack, Adrian. *Carnivorous plants.* Cambridge, MA; The MIT Press. 1979.

Walkup, Crystal. *Index of Species Information: Sarracenia Purpurea.* At: *fs.fed.us/database/feis/plants/forb/sarpur/all.html.* 1991.

uptodate.com/*contents/epidemiology-clinical-manifestations-and-diagnosis-of-genital-herpes-simplex-virus-infection*

webmd.com/*vitamins-supplements/ingredientmono-103-PITCHER%20PLANT.aspx?activeIngredientId=103&activeIngredientName=PITCHER%20PLAN*

Appendix B

Summary of Case Studies

Abstract: *Sarracenia purpurea* (pitcher plant) was discovered in the 1800s as a remedy for small pox (Chalmers 1862). Since this time, however, it has received no accolades as a treatment for viral or any other condition, being thought of as medically "obsolete" (LaGow 2004).

A compounded formulation of the pitcher plant extract in an aloe vera derived *Gel (Gowey Protocol® Gel)* was applied topically to various patient lesions known to be "therapeutic challenges" (Bacelieri and Johnson 2005): squamous cell carcinoma, Kaposi's sarcoma, cervical dysplasia, herpes simplex virus, methicillin-resistant staphylococcus aureus (MRSA), and plantar warts.

All patients receiving treatment of this compounded formulation showed rapid benefit and a complete resolution of symptoms (as presented clinically or via pre and post lab results).

Introduction: According to Colgan et al. (2003) "viral infections are among the formidable conditions in the primary care setting, carrying a wide range of illnesses that are difficult to treat". Viruses plus diseases, such as MRSA or dysplastic cells, create challenges for any practitioner and are aggravated by high stress levels, compromised immune systems, nutrient deficiency, and low socioeconomic statuses (Bower, Palmieri and Dhillon 2006).

A compounded formulation, termed the "*Gowey Protocol® Gel*", of the pitcher plant was made for the author by Professional Compounding Centers of America

(PCCA) in a base derived from aloe vera. The *Gowey Protocol®Gel* was applied directly to patient lesions with appropriate follow-up.

Methods: Patients were given the *Gowey Protocol® Gel*, and applied the formulation topically to lesions every three to four hours and in the cervical dysplasia case, nightly (inserted via a vaginal applicator). Patients were followed up with daily or weekly, per informed consent, from 2009-2011.

Results

MRSA: A five-year-old male with a history of repeat MRSA lesions, presented to the office with recent outbreaks diagnosed via lab cultures. MRSA was on the lateral aspects of the patient's hands and feet bilaterally.

Patient was prescribed the *Gowey Protocol® Gel* to be applied every three to four hours. Within 24 hours, lesions were clearing up and, within two days, were completely gone upon objective inspection. No post culture was obtained, per patient preference.

Plantar warts: Patient presented with a plantar wart located on the heel of her left foot. She was given the *Gowey Protocol® Gel* and instructed to cover the wart with a bandage. Warts scabbed over within four weeks and were gone by six weeks. Pre- and post-biopsy was not obtained, per patient preference.

Kaposi's sarcoma: Patient experiences Kaposi's sarcoma as ulcerations on lower extremities, which are very painful. *Gowey Protocol® Gel* was applied around and on top of current lesions that were newly erupting. Pain dissipated immediately and over the course of a few days, prevented ulcerations from deepening to the bone (clinical observation).

Herpes simplex: Patient presented with new, 10/10 painful herpes vesicles (5), located on the labia majora bilaterally. Diagnosis was confirmed with positive blood titer for HSV II by another physician. *Gowey Protocol® Gel* was applied directly to the vesicles every three to four hours; lesions were healed (clinical observation) within three days.

Cervical Dysplasia: Patient with low-grade squamous cell carcinoma intraepithelial lesion of the cervical epithelium presented to the clinic requesting alternative treatment. Author applied the *Gowey Protocol® Gel* to the cervix bimonthly and instructed the patient to inserted nightly, with a vaginal applicator. Patient received a follow-up pap within six months and results were within normal limits.

Squamous cell carcinoma: Patient presented with a new lesion that was not healing on the left lateral aspect of her nose. Biopsy results revealed squamous cell carcinoma; patient scheduled for Moh's but requested treatment regardless. She was prescribed the **Gowey Protocol® Gel** to be applied every three to four hours. Lesions began to heal within one week; Moh's was cancelled due to normal biopsy on follow-up visit one month later.

Discussion

These series of cases demonstrate the possible effectiveness of the pitcher plant in treating a variety of conditions. Further clinical trials, with pre- and post-labs, skin cultures or biopsies need to be done to confirm efficacy of *S. purpurea* when treating topical skin conditions.

The **Gowey Protocol® Gel** base needs to be studied so as to remove chance that the base itself is contributing to the mechanism of healing. It is possible that because of the action of anthocyanins within the pitcher plant that apoptosis of damaged cells is the contributory factor in healing (Sheridan 2001).

References

Bacelieri, Rocky and Johnson, Sandra J. *Cutaneous Warts: An Evidence-Based Approach to Therapy.* **American Family Physicians.** 2005. 72(4): 647-652.

Bower M, Palmieri C, Dhillon T. *AIDS and related malignancies; changing epidemiology and the impact era of highly active anti-retroviral therapy.* **Current Opinion in Infectious Diseases.** 2006. 19: 14-19.

Chalmers, Miles. *The Employment of Sarracenia Purpurea, or Indian Pitcher Plant as a Remedy for Small Pox.* **The Lancet.** 1862. p 430-431.

Colgan, Richard et al. *Antiviral drugs in the immunocompetent host: part one, treatment of hepatitis, cytomegalovirus, and herpes infections.* **American Family Physicians.** 2003. 67(4): 757-762.

LaGow, Bette. **PDR for Herbal Medicines.** Thompson; Montvale, NJ. 2004.

Sheridan, PM and Griesbach, RJ. *Anthocyanins of Sarracenia L Flowers and Leaves.* **Hort Science** 2001. 36(2): 384.

Williams, RJ et al. *Flavanoids, antioxidants, and signaling molecules.* **Free Radical Biology and Medicine.** 2004. 36(7): 838-49.

Appendix C

Supplements

I have been working with supplements and supplement companies since my early-twenties (a long time ago!). I got my start while working for Whole Foods Market in Madison, Wisconsin. My knowledge of supplements deepened when I got to Naturopathic medical school, and especially when I started to prescribe for patients.

Unfortunately, many if not most supplements do not absorb well. Many supplements are bought because they are cheap or because of good marketing techniques, not necessarily because they are good products yielding good results. My products (Mother Nature's Remedy) are formulated with absorption in mind. The following companies have products that are formulated with that in mind as well, or have excellent quality standards. You can find a sampling of these products on my website, *howdoitreatnaturally.com*.

Supplement companies I endorse include:

- • *Integrative Therapeutics*
- • *Thorne*
- • *Seroyal*
- • *Biopharmica*
- • *Xymogen*
- • *Mountain Peaks Nutritionals*

Thank you for supporting me in my efforts. I also know that, some day, I will build a Naturopathic Hospital. With your help financially, I will be able to accomplish that.

Appendix D

Becoming a Patient

I treat patients from around the country, via phone consultations. If you do not live in Flagstaff, Arizona, and cannot see me in person, you may schedule a phone consultation. My intake form is available online at *naturopathsinternational.org*.

My office number is 928.214.8793.

I have been working with plants since I was in my early teens, and became a Botanist and Conservation Biologist through my time in college. I graduated from the University of Wisconsin-Madison in 1999, then went on to medical school in 2003. I attended the Southwest College of Naturopathic Medicine in Tempe, AZ.

Upon graduation I founded Naturopaths International (NI, *naturopathsinternational. org*), went to Nepal to volunteer in domestic violence shelters for Saathi (*saathi.org*), then came back to Arizona to start NI's first clinic. I focused on building NI's clinic while volunteering my time in domestic violence shelters throughout Arizona. I went back to Nepal three times to volunteer for the Saathi, and engaged other physicians in serving with me.

Since that time I started a mobile medical outreach branch of NI, took a group of physicians to Haiti after the 2010 earthquake, and worked with our volunteer physicians to provide over a million dollars in free services and medical supplies to patients in need. We have had to cut back on our free outreach due to lack of funding.

I hope to get those programs going again from the sales of this book.

Thank you!

References

Aihara, Herman. *Acid and Alkaline*. George Ohsawa Macrobiotic Foundation; Oroville, CA. 1986.

Anderson, Sonja et al. *Detection of gene amplification of the human telomerase gene TERC, a potential marker for triage of women with HPV positive abnormal pap smears. Am J Pathol*. 2009. Nov; 175(5): 1831-1847.

Basu J et al. *Plasma uric acid levels in women with cervical intraepithelial neoplasia. **Nutr Cancer***. 2005. 51(1): 25-31.

Bi pin, Sawani et al. *Increased risk of cervical dysplasia in long-term survivors of allogenic stem cell transplantation: implications for screening and HPV vaccinations. **Biol Blood Marrow Transplant***. 2010. Sept 7.

Chatterjee, Korshik et al. *CCR2-V641 polymorphism is associated with increased risk of cervical cancer but not with HPV infection or pre-cancerous lesions. **BMC Cancer***. 2010. 10: 2778.

Chichareon, SB and Tocharoenvanish S. *Risk factors of having high-grade cervical intraepithelial neoplasia/invasive carcinoma in women with vaginal glandular cells of undetermined significant smears. **Int Journal of Gynecol Cancer***. 2006. Mar-April; 16(2): 56-74.

Cho H et al. *Relationship of serum antioxidant micronutrients and sociodemograhic factors to cervical neoplasia, a case-control study. **Clin Chem Lab Med***. 2009. 47(8): 1005-12.

Crinnion, Walter, NMD. *Do Environmental Toxicants Contribute to Allergy and Asthma? **Alternative Medicine Review***. 2012. Vol 17, No 1.

Crinnion, Walter, NMD. *Long-term effects of chronic low dose mercury exposure*. 2003.

Crinnion, Walter, NMD. *Mechanism of Defense: protection, biotransformation, excretion.* 2003.

Crinnion, Walter, NMD. *Role of macronutrients in biotransformation.* 2003.

Crinnion, Walter, NMD. *Lectures on naturopathic environmental detox.* Southwest College of Naturopathic Medicine, Tempe, AZ. 2005 lecture series.

Dossey, Larry, MD. **Healing Words**. Harper; New York, NY. 1993.

Emedicinehealth.com

Epstein, RJ. *Primary prevention of human papillomavirus dependent neoplasia: no condom, no sex.* **Eur J. Cancer**. 2005. Nov; 71(17): 2, 595-600.

Dennis F, Hanz S, Alain S. *Clearance, persistence, and recurrance of HPV infection.* **Gynecol, Obstet, Fertil.** 2008. Apr; 36(4): 430-40.

Fang, Carolyn. *Perceived Stress is Associated with Impaired T-cell response to HPV 16 in Women with Cervical Dysplasia.* **Annual of Behavior Medicine**. 2008. February; 35(1): 87-96.

Fenseca et al. *Smoking and cervical cancer.* **ISRN Obstet Gynecol.** 2011. 847-684.

Firnhaber, Cynthia. *Diversely high prevalence of HPV associated with a significant high rate of cervical dysplasia in HIV infected women in Johannesburg, South Africa.* **Acta Cytol.** 2009. Jan-Feb; 53(1); 10-17.

Flatley JE et al. *Folate status and aberrant DNA methylation are associated with HPV infection and cervical pathogenesis.* **Cancer Epidemiol Biomarkers Prev.** 2009. Oct; 18(10): 2782-9.

Gaines, MM; Schwinge PJ, Fortney JA. *Depo medroxyprogesterone acetate and combined oral contraceptive and cervical cancer in-situ in women aged 50 years or younger.* **West Indian Med J.** 2004. Dec; 53(6): 406-12.

Goodman, MT et al. *CYP1A1, GSTM1, GSST polymorphism and the risk of cervical squamous cell intraepithelial lesions in multiethinic populations.* **Gynecol Oncol.** 2001. May; 81(2): 263-9.

Greenspan, Francis and Strewler, Gordon. **Basic and Clinical Endocrinology**. Appleton and Lange, Stamford, CT; 1997.

Hefler, L et al. *Treatment with vaginal progesterone in women with low grade cervical dysplasia; a phase II trial.* **Anticancer Research.** 2010. Apr; 30(4): 1257-61.

Hernandez BY et al. *Reports: plasma and dietary phytoestrogens and risk of premalignant lesions of the cervix.* **Nut Cancer.** 2004; 44(2): 109-24.

Kato, R; Chiesara E; Vasanelli, P. *Factors influencing induction of hepatic microsomal drug metabolizing enzymes.* **Biochem Pharmacol.** 1962. 11; 211-220.

Kihara, Takashi et al. *Repeated sauna treatment improves vascular endothelial and cardiac function in patietns with chronic heart failure.* **Journal of the American College of Cardiology**. 2002. Vol 39, No. 5; 774-759.

Kim SY et al. *Changes in Lipid peroxidation and antioxidant trace elements in serum of women with cervical intraepithelial neoplasia and invasive cancer.* **Nutr Cancer**. 2003. 47(2): 126-30.

Kneipp, Sebastian. **My Water Cure**. Pilgrims Book, Delhi. 1998 reprint.

Kwanbunjan K, et al. *Vitamin B12 status of Thai women with neoplasia of the cervic uterui.* **SE Asian J Trop Med**. 2006. 37 Suppl; 3:178-83.

Lee GJ et al. *Antioxidant liquid peroxidation in patients with cervical intraepithelial neoplasia.* **J Korean Med Sci**. 2005. Apr; 20(2): 267-72.

Lehtinen M, et al. *Overall efficacy of HPV 16/18 ASo4 adjuvanted vaccine against grade 3 or greater cervical intraepithelial neoplasia: 4 year end-of-study analysis of the randomized, double-blind PATRICIA trial.* **Lancet Oncol**. 2012. Jan 13(1); 89-99.

Liv T et al. *A case control study of nutritional factors and cervical dysplasia.* **Cancer Epidemiol Biomarkers Prev**. 1993. Nov-Dec; 2(6): 525-30.

LuK'uan, Yu. **Taoist Yoga**. Samual Weiser, Inc., York Beach, Maine. 1973.

Marshall, K et al. *Dietary nutrients low in women with cervical dysplasia.* 2003-2005. At Lef.org/protocols/femals_reproductive/cervical_dysplasia.02htm.

McFarlane-Anderson, Normal et al. *Cervical Dysplasia and Cancer and the Use of Hormonal Contraceptives in Jamacian Women.* **BMC Health**. 2008. 8: 9.

Mdconsult.com

Medscape.com

Mesher, D et al. *Long-term follow up in cervical disease in women screened by cytology and HPV testing; results from the HART study.* **Br J Cancer**. 2010. Apr 27; 102(9): 1405-1410.

Moodley M et al. *The role of steroid conraceptive hormones in the pathogenesis of invasive cervical cancer: a review.* **Integrative Journal of Gynecol Cancer.** 2003. May-April; 13(2): 103-10.

Nlm.nih.gov

Osteen, Joel. **Your Best Life Now**. Warner Faith, New York, NY. 2005.

Powell, Dirk WM. **Endocrinology and Naturopatic Therapies**. Department of Natural Medicine, Bastyr University; Bothell, WA. 2004.

Reich, O and Regaver, S. *CK17 and p16 expression patterns distinguish atypical immature squamous metaplasia from high-grade cervical intraepithelial neoplasia (CINII).* **Histopathology.** 2007. 50: 629-635.

Reich, O. *Is early first intercourse a risk factor for cervical cancer?* **Gynekol Guburtshilfiche Rundsch.** 2005. Oct; 45(4): 251-6.

Samir, R, et al. *Oral Contraceptive and progestin-only use correlates to tissue marker expression in women with cervical intraepithelial neoplasia.* **Contraception.** 2011. Oct 11.

Salazar EL et al. *Influence of the use of oral contraceptives as risk factors for human papillomavirus infection and cervical intraepithelial neoplasia.* **Gynecol Obstet Mex.** 2005. Feb; 73(2): 83-9.

Sanson, SL et al. *The effect of loop electrosurgical excision procedure on future pregnancy outcomes.* **Obstet and gynecol.** 2005. Feb; 105(2): 325-32.

Seresini, Samantha et al. *DC4+ T cells against HPV-18 E7 in patients with high-grade cervical lesions associated with the abnormal sense of the virus in the cervix.* **Immunology.** 2010. Sept; 131(1): 89-98.

Sheridan, PM and Griesbach, RJ. *Anthocyanins of Sarracenia L Flowers and Leaves.* **Hort Science** 2001. 36(2): 384.

Skaper SD, Giusti P, Facci L. *Microglia and mast cells: two tracks on the road to neuroinflammation.* **FASEB J.** 2012. Apr 19.

Tomita LY et al. *Diet and serum micronutrients in relation to cervical neoplasia and cancer among low-income Brazilian women.* **Int J Cancer.** 2010. Feb 1; 126(3): 703-14.

Tolstrup J et al. *The role of smoking and alcohol intake in the development of high-grade squamous intraepithelial lesios among high risk HPV positive women.* **Acta Obstet Gynecol Scand.** 2006. 85(9): 1114-9.

Tong SY et al. *Functional polymorphism in manganese superoxide dismutase and antioxidant status: their interactions or the risk of cervical intraepithelial neoplasia and cervical cancer.* **Gynecol Oncol.** 2009. Nov; 115(2): 272-6.

Trimble, Cornelia et al. *Spontaneous Regression of High-Grade Cervical Dysplasia: effects of Human Papillomavirus Type HLA Phenotype.* Clinical **Cancer Research.** 2005. July 1; 91(3): 4717-4728.

Umm.edu/altmed/articles/cervical-dysplasia-000034.htm

Virtue, Doreen. **Angel Words.** Hay House; Carlesbad, CA. 2010.

Watrous, Letitia, ND. *Constitutional Hydrotherapy: from nature cure to advanced naturopathic medicine.* **Journal of Natural Medicine.** 1998. 7(2): 72-78.

Xiocheng, Wu et al. *Human Papillomavirus—Associated Cancers—United States, 2004-2008.* ***Morbidity and Mortality Weekly Report.*** 2012. 61(15): 258-261.

Zbroch T et al. *Lifestyle, chlymydia, trachomatis infection, bacterial vaginosis, and their impact on the frequency of cervical lesions.* ***Ginekol Pol.*** 2004. Jul; 75: 538-44.

CPSIA information can be obtained at www.ICGtesting.com
Printed in the USA
LVOW01s1728211113

362270LV00017B/55/P

9 781614 486848